AF885231

The Complete Guide To

VIRECHANA

Dr. Jessica Vellela, BAMS

&

Dr. Prasanth Dharmarajan, PhD (Āyu)

To be used under direct supervision of an

ĀYURVEDA ĀCHĀRYA (qualified Āyurvedic Doctor)

in holistic & sustainable Āyurvedic healthcare

ĀYU Academy
1001 South Main Street, Suite 500
Kalispell, MT 59901
https://www.ayu.academy

The Complete Guide To Virechana

First Edition

Authors

Dr. Jessica Vellela, BAMS
Dr. Prasanth Dharmarajan, PhD (Ayu)

Copyright © 2022 by ĀYU Academy LLC
All Rights Reserved.

No part of this publication may be reproduced, utilized or transmitted in any form by any means, including electronic, mechanical, photocopying, recording or storage by any information system or retrieval device, without the written permission of the publisher.

ISBN: 978-1-950876-17-4

Notice – Disclaimer

Knowledge and best practices in the field of Āyurveda have been well-established, continuously practiced scientifically and documented in Sanskrit for at least 2,000 years in India and neighboring countries. Information included in this manual is based on established and current best practices in India today. Permissible adaptations are included only where they adhere to the scientific principles and application of Āyurvedic medical protocols. Every effort has been made to ensure that the content provided in this publication is accurate and complete at the time of publishing. However, this is not an exhaustive treatment of the subject. No liability is assumed for personal harm, injury, medical complications, losses or damages due to the information provided. Interpretation and application of information from this publication is solely the responsibility of the reader. Always consult a qualified professional for personal healthcare needs.

Do not use this publication for self-treatment.

The Complete Guide To Virechana should only be used under direct supervision of an Āyurveda Āchārya (Āyurvedic Doctor), qualified to practice Āyurvedic medicine in India, Sri Lanka or Nepal.

नगरी नगरस्येव रथस्येव रथी यथा ।
स्वशरीरस्य मेधावी कृत्येष्ववहितो भवेत् ।।१०३।।

च. सू. ५।१०३

Nagarī nagarasyeva rathasyeva rathī yathā |
Svaśharīrasya medhāvī kṛtyeṣhvavahito bhavet || 103 ||

Cha. Sū. 5/103

Just as a city's protector or a chariot's driver are ever vigilant,
an intelligent person should remain proactive in caring for their own body.

Wishing all beings

harmonious health

for a lifetime

and beyond

How to use this book

If you're getting ready to read this book, you might be preparing for one of Āyurveda's best opportunities to create personal, sustainable health, a medical Pañcha Karma procedure called Virechana (pronounced "vih-RAY-chuh-nuh"). This is a complex procedure that must be customized and performed under supervision of a qualified* Āyurveda Āchārya.

Use this book to learn about the process, options and requirements as you research Virechana to consider whether it may be appropriate for you. Pay close attention to the details of each stage, time requirements and restrictions in diet and activities.

If you decide to work with an Āyurveda Āchārya to go through Virechana for yourself, use this book as a guide throughout the process. The Appendices contain preparation checklists and daily journals to record key pieces of information. These records will help you continue to learn and understand the process for months and years to come through changes you experience. They also provide valuable support for any future Pañcha Karma procedures.

Virechana is a powerful procedure and inherently poses risk, especially in complex cases. Please make certain that you are under direct care and guidance of a qualified* Āyurveda Āchārya who knows you well and can care for you properly for at least several weeks before, during and after the procedure.

To learn more about Āyurveda and to find a qualified* Āyurveda Āchārya, please visit http://www.myayu.com.

*Qualified refers to a graduate of accredited, Āyurvedic medical training in India, Nepal or Sri Lanka who is licensed to practice Āyurvedic medicine.

Scientific foundations and evidence

Information presented in this book is based on the classical science of Āyurvedic medicine as it is practiced in India today. Additional information from Western sciences and biomedicine is included to explain human physiology in familiar terms.

Evidence for safety and efficacy of Āyurvedic medicine exists in India today largely through continuous practice in long-standing educational and research institutions, hospitals and clinics. Much of this evidence is contained in Indian languages including Sanskrit, Malayalam and Hindi, through written and oral practices. Contemporary evidence is growing, but it will likely take several years or decades for peer-reviewed, scientific literature to become well-established in English.

The inherent complexity of Āyurveda would be best suited for research, testing and proof using an evidence-based framework that aligns with its structure. At the time of this writing, no such testing structure exists. Western biomedical models and standards can be used, but they require significant translation in framework and terminology. This confusion casts doubt on the efficacy and validity of Āyurveda and contributes to its reputation as a pseudoscience in some spheres.

Āyurveda has served as a robust, complete health care system for millennia. An estimated 70% of India's rural population depends on Āyurvedic medicine today[1].

On a global level, it is imperative that scientific practices of Āyurvedic medicine be available to those who want to use them. This publication intends to provide access to these practices in their authentic, complex, scientific form for those who voluntarily choose to employ them for personal health.

---

[1] Pandey MM, Rastogi S, Rawat AK. Indian traditional ayurvedic system of medicine and nutritional supplementation. Evid Based Complement Alternat Med. 2013;2013:376327. doi: 10.1155/2013/376327. Epub 2013 Jun 23. PMID: 23864888; PMCID: PMC3705899.

Use of Sanskrit for Āyurvedic medical terms

Sanskrit terms used in this book come directly from classical literature of Āyurvedic medicine. Sanskrit is formatted throughout this book as follows.

Italicization Sanskrit terms are italicized except for common words that exist in the English dictionary (like Āyurveda) or that are used repeatedly throughout this book (like Virechana, or Pañcha Karma).

Anglicization Sanskrit terms are Anglicized throughout this book. When using Sanskrit terms, they may be modified to fit the sentence using proper English grammatical rules. English plural endings will use "-es" for terms ending in "s" (example, singular *srotas* [a network of channels] with plural *srotases*). Apostrophes indicate possession (example, The three *doṣhas'* behavior is complex.). The first letter of the term is capitalized at the beginning of a sentence. These changes do not alter the original meaning or indicate differences in the meaning of the original Sanskrit terms.

Diacritics Sanskrit terms often contain accent marks, dots and other additions to Latin script (letters). These are called diacritical marks, or diacritics, and they indicate specific pronunciation methods for Sanskrit sounds. Diacritics are required for lossless matching to the original, 49-syllable, Sanskrit alphabet. Placement of diacritical marks is based on standardized systems of transliteration.

Transliteration scheme This book uses the Āyurvedic Universal Transliteration Scheme (ĀYUT) to represent single Sanskrit phonetic sounds with Latin letters using diacritical marks. The 49 sounds of the Sanskrit alphabet are matched one-to-one to an expanded Latin alphabet with added diacritics.

The Complete Guide To Virechana

Table of Contents

Chapter 1: Virechana and Medical Pañcha Karma

Virechana (pronounced "vih-RAY-chuh-nuh") is one of five powerful therapeutic procedures in Āyurvedic medicine in the practice of Pañcha Karma (pronounced "punch-uh KAH-r-muh") that is capable of managing, curing and preventing disease.

Pañcha Karma, also transliterated or spelled Pañchakarma, or Pañcakarma (with IAST transliteration), is a group of five complex, bio-purification procedures in Āyurvedic medicine that are designed to eliminate accumulated metabolic wastes from the physical body. Each of the five procedures is a primer for subsequent regenerative protocols in Āyurvedic medicine.

The phrase "Pañcha Karma" consists of two Sanskrit terms.

Pañcha	Pañcha means the number five.
Karma	Karma refers to a therapeutic procedure in the context of Āyurvedic medicine.

In general use, the Sanskrit word *karma* refers to any action. In the context of Āyurvedic medicine, *karma* indicates the specific actions performed to achieve the two main goals of Āyurveda, to maintain health and cure disease.

All five of the Pañcha Karma procedures remove physical waste from the human body and attempt to restore the normal, baseline state. These methods of bio-purification aid the body in eliminating debris and pollutants from tissues, organs and channels which are often locked in deep fat storage systems.

Even the healthiest people naturally experience varying amounts of waste buildup in their bodies over the course of normal life. These accumulated waste products are called *doṣhas* (pronounced "DOH-shuhs"). *Doṣhas* are a complex concept in Āyurvedic medicine that refers to both waste materials and the foundational building blocks of robust health.

Doṣhas should be understood to behave as physiological switches that signal instructions to create disease or health, based on their inputs. They are controlled by myriad internal and external factors including genetics, epigenetics, environment, diet, lifestyle, thoughts and emotions (through neurotransmitters), circadian rhythm, sleep and wake cycles, and more. Essentially, *doṣhas* are an individual's tendency toward a particular state of being. They are often closely related to the triggers that dysregulate normal, healthy functions. A good example of a *doṣhic* flare would be an allergic reaction to specific foods like dairy, sugar or gluten.

Once the *doṣhas* are switched into a dysfunctional state, they initiate and promote dysregulation and degeneration of normal functions, contributing to the development of disease. With correct management in Āyurvedic medicine, these switches can be restored to their normal, healthy positions to halt disease processes and allow the body to regenerate health.

Āyurvedic medicine defines the three *doṣhas* of the physical body: *vāta*, *pitta* and *kapha*. Each is primarily located in a home location or "seat" and is responsible for regulation of a host of functions. *Vāta* is located in the lower portion of the body, from the navel downwards, and primarily seated in the large intestines. *Pitta* is located in the middle portion of the body, from the base of the sternum to the navel, and primarily seated in the small intestines. *Kapha* is located in the upper portion of the body, from the sternum upwards, and primarily seated in the lungs and chest.

Doṣhas are understood to be in a constant state of flux based on causative factors from nourishment, rest, environment, season, stress, psychological state, and more. The changes can cause a *doṣha* to remain within its normal range of upper and lower boundaries, reduce and become deficient, or increase and become accumulated or excessive. Based on specific signs and symptoms of an individual's presentation, an Āyurveda Āchārya is able to assess and diagnose current states of *doṣhas* and progression of disease to determine an appropriate treatment plan.

Digestion and metabolism play a key role in the normal and abnormal functions of the *doṣhas*. Āyurvedic medicine explains digestion and metabolism under the concept of *agni* (pronounced "ugh-nee").

Agni is like the body's energy-producing motor and is responsible for conversion of all consumed foods and drinks into usable energy. Many factors reduce or inhibit strong, healthy functioning of *agni*. The most common causes of dysregulated digestion and metabolism include:

- Eating too much at once
- Eating too frequently, before the previous meal has digested
- Eating combinations of foods that do not digest well together
- Eating the wrong things, especially at the wrong times
- Engaging in any activities or emotions that inhibit or impair digestion

When *agni* is functioning sub-optimally, its conversion processes produce metabolic waste called *āma* (pronounced "AH-muh"). The *doṣhas* can further complicate this by congealing with *āma* to scatter throughout the body. These waste materials clog macro and micro channels, disrupt physiological functions and lead to the development of acute and chronic disease.

The goal of Pañcha Karma and Virechana is to expel accumulated waste materials from the body in a controlled fashion. These waste materials must be safely sequestered and escorted out of the body without creating side effects, complications or secondary diseases.

Each of the five procedures in Pañcha Karma targets a specific *doṣha* in its primary home location in the physical body to facilitate its elimination from the nearest route of anatomical exit. Virechana is the second of five procedures in Pañcha Karma and its primary mode of action is to eliminate excess *pitta doṣha* from the small intestines downward through the lower portion of the digestive tract and rectum. This effectively produces a hard reset of digestion and metabolism and likely slows or perhaps reverses some biological aging processes.

Virechana is one of the more complex Pañcha Karma procedures because of its sequential staging and the mechanics required to change physiology in a living human being. It temporarily reverses the body's normal activities of waste development and storage, and clears the pathways to activate regeneration.

The term Virechana is a technical Sanskrit term used in Āyurvedic Medicine. It combines the prefix *"vi-"* with the root term *"rechana"* to indicate a process which methodically and systematically eliminates waste materials as *doṣhas* from the body through the lower route (ie, the rectal passage) via purgation, or bowel movements.

Out of the five therapeutic procedures in Pañcha Karma, Virechana is the one which generally provides the best results with the lowest risk, stress and discomfort compared to other procedures. It is an intense procedure and must be conducted under direct supervision of an Āyurveda Āchārya, or Vaidya, who is an Āyurvedic Doctor trained at an accredited institution in India, Nepal or Sri Lanka with minimum qualification of BAMS (Bachelor of Āyurvedic Medicine and Surgery).

The medical practice of Virechana can be performed in two ways, based on classical instructions.

Complete Virechana	Mini Virechana
• More complex • Longer duration (17 to 25 days) • Stronger, long-lasting, positive effects	• Less complex • Shorter duration (5 to 11 days) • Weaker, short-term, positive effects

Both formats must be completed in their entirety. Virechana cannot be interrupted once started. It is important to plan well and be fully aware of all requirements, time commitments and other demands when considering doing Virechana.

For almost every person who undergoes this therapeutic procedure, there are moments of doubt and regret due to physical, mental and emotional discomfort. These moments are key indicators of the correct functioning of the process and must be tolerated. Certain signs and symptoms of discomfort are expected and may indicate the separation of accumulated waste materials (*doṣhas*) from the physical body. After being safely dislodged via lubrication, waste materials can be mobilized and directed to the gastro-intestinal tract. Then they are methodically expelled through bowel movements.

For several weeks to months following Complete Virechana, positive results typically continue to manifest. This is when most people recognize that even the most severe moments of discomfort during the process are worth the benefits.

The five medical Pañcha Karma procedures include

1. Vamana	Therapeutic emesis
2. Virechana	Therapeutic purgation
3. Basti (two types)	Therapeutic enema
a. Nirūha	Emulsion enema
b. Anuvāsana	Oil enema
4. Nasya	Therapeutic nasal instillation
5. Rakta mokṣhaṇa	Therapeutic blood-letting

Pañcha Karma is like performing surgical operations on the body without the tools that require physical incision, extraction, probing or other methods. When done properly, Pañcha Karma eliminates a significant load of accumulated waste materials (as *doṣhas*), it resets digestion and metabolism (*agni*), it restores normal, healthy physiological function of the body and mind and it activates regeneration. It provides a powerful opportunity to learn how the body works, better recognize abnormal, unhealthy function and experience normal, healthy function in a relatively short period of time.

However, these powerful effects and outcomes also carry high risk. Medical Pañcha Karma is generally best performed in an Āyurvedic medical facility in a country like India, Nepal or Sri Lanka under direct supervision of a qualified Āyurveda Āchārya, or Āyurvedic Doctor, who has completed a minimum level of training of the Bachelor's of Āyurvedic Medicine and Surgery (BAMS).

All Pañcha Karma practices must have backup and emergency medical plans in place. At a minimum, this involves planned transfer to a nearby medical facility capable of managing common complications like dehydration, anaphylaxis and allergic reactions like uncontrollable vomiting or diarrhea. Properly-equipped centers will have nurses, medical doctors, medical supplies and equipment on site.

In most countries, Āyurveda and Pañcha Karma are largely unregulated and almost anyone can advertise or claim that they are providing these services. Always do thorough research and carefully evaluate potential practitioners.

Complete vs Mini Pañcha Karma

Complete and Mini Pañcha Karma differ in their time requirements, efficacy and expected clinical outcomes. When used at the right time for individual conditions, each can be highly effective.

Complete Pañcha Karma generally requires several weeks to perform protocols that produce, deeper physiological changes with stronger, long-term, positive improvements. Multiple applications of Complete Pañcha Karma can often reverse and cure a wide range of diseases.

Mini Pañcha Karma can often be completed at home under supervision of a qualified Āyurveda Āchārya in a few days with significantly less interruption to one's regular, daily life. Even though it can only produce limited, brief, positive improvements, it may still be beneficial for maintenance when Complete Pañcha Karma is not available. It also is an excellent initial procedure for those who want to test an easier Pañcha Karma experience on themselves before committing to a Complete Virechana.

Because of the complexity of Complete Pañcha Karma, it is best performed in an established Āyurvedic medical facility under 24/7 supervision. This provides a properly controlled environment with access to a full range of treatments, medicines and care required for the planned procedure, as well as the expertise needed to manage any unforeseen complications that may arise. While this is the best option, it presents numerous challenges with travel, time zone changes, food, cultural adjustment and unpredictable costs.

Outside India, Pañcha Karma is almost always diluted, unscientific and unsafe. Lack of global regulation of Āyurveda has resulted in heavy commercialization of select treatments that incorrectly represent the classical medical practices of Complete Pañcha Karma. These spa practices are called Pañcha Karma Lite and they are often heavily marketed as relaxing, comforting experiences. True, medical Pañcha Karma is rarely easy or enjoyable. Most would consider it intense, hard work.

When performed properly, medical Pañcha Karma is able to reverse disease and significantly bolster baseline health. In India today, it is regularly used to treat a wide variety of complex, acute and chronic conditions. It also acts as a preventive measure to create and maintain optimal states of personalized health especially when used with correct, ongoing diet and lifestyle activities.

Classically, medical Pañcha Karma is recommended to be performed each year during middle age (approximately 12 to 70 years) in the appropriate season as a preventive measure. As a treatment for disease, it can be performed more frequently, and in younger and older individuals as appropriate to the individual case. One or more procedures may be indicated in sequence, based on time available, disease progression and other factors.

Only a qualified Āyurveda Āchārya can properly assess, diagnose, recommend and oversee medical Pañcha Karma. The determination for medical Pañcha Karma is based on an individual's personal history, complete medical history, current presentation and limitations (time, finances, commitments, etc). In India, certain treatments within the scope of Pañcha Karma are used for emergency management. Typically, Indian patients can undergo Pañcha Karma with one to four weeks of advance notice because of compatible dietary habits and other accustomed factors.

Outside India, however, Complete Pañcha Karma requires anywhere from one to six months of preparation and education to ensure a safe experience and successful outcome. The correct application of Complete Pañcha Karma outside India is fully capable of reversing disease, resetting baseline health and acting as a strong preventive measure. This requires several months of time, attention, discipline and compliance before, during and after the procedure to ensure a successful outcome.

Compare options for Complete Pañcha Karma and Mini Pañcha Karma next.

Complete Pañcha Karma	Can be performed	
Procedure	At an Āyurvedic medical facility	At home, under an Āyurveda Āchārya
Vamana Therapeutic emesis	Yes	No
Days required	Min 15 days	N/A
Virechana Therapeutic purgation	Yes	Yes, select cases
Days required	Min 17 days	Min 14 days
Basti Therapeutic enema	Yes	No
Days required	Min 4 or 8 days	N/A
Nasya Therapeutic nasal instillation	Yes	Yes, select cases
Days required	Min 7 days	Min 3 days
Rakta mokṣhaṇa Therapeutic bloodletting	Yes	No
Days required	Min 3 treatments	N/A

Mini Pañcha Karma	**Can be performed**	
Procedure	At an Āyurvedic medical facility	At home, under an Āyurveda Āchārya
Mini Vamana Therapeutic emesis	Yes	Yes, select cases
Days required	Min 4 days	Min 4 days
Mini Virechana Therapeutic purgation	Yes	Yes, select cases
Days required	Min 5 days	Min 5 days
Mini Basti Therapeutic enema	Yes	Yes, select cases Only 1 type of basti
Days required	Min 3 days	Min 3 days
Mini Nasya Therapeutic nasal instillation	Yes	Yes, select cases
Days required	Min 3 days	Min 3 days
Mini Rakta mokṣhana Therapeutic bloodletting	Yes	Yes, select cases
Days required	Min 3 days	Min 3 days

Comparing Pañcha Karma options

The main options for Pañcha Karma include

Complete Pañcha Karma – Also called Medical Pañcha Karma, or Classical Pañcha Karma

- Long, intense, deep procedures that produce long-term, positive improvements
- Safest when performed in an Āyurvedic medical facility
- At home options only available for Virechana and Nasya
- At home application available on a case-by-case basis, under supervision of a qualified Āyurveda Āchārya

Mini Pañcha Karma

- Shorter, easier procedures with limited positive improvements
- Most are safe to be performed at home under supervision of a qualified Āyurveda Āchārya

Spa Pañcha Karma – Also called Pañcha Karma Lite

- For relaxation and beauty
- Not capable of producing targeted, therapeutic outcomes

These details are summarized and compared in the following table.

	Medical, or Complete, or Classical Pañcha Karma	Mini Pañcha Karma	Spa Pañcha Karma or Pañcha Karma Lite
Where it can be performed	• Āyurvedic medical facility • Limited options at home for select cases	• Āyurvedic medical facility • At home	• Āyurvedic medical facility • At home • Resort, wellness center
Requires supervision	Yes, Āyurveda Āchārya	Yes, Āyurveda Āchārya	Yes, Āyurveda Āchārya, but unregulated practice allows otherwise which increases risk
Risk level	High	Moderate	Low
Expected therapeutic effect	• Eliminates deep *doṣhas* • Resolves root cause • Cures disease	• Eliminates superficial *doṣhas* • Pacifies and reduces disease	• Adjunct therapies for superficial relaxation
Treatments available	Complete • Vamana • Virechana • Basti (2 types) • Nasya • Rakta mokṣhaṇa	Mini • Vamana • Virechana • Basti (1 type) • Nasya • Upakrama (adjunct physical treatments)	Physical treatments • Massages • Sweat induction • Pouring (head, body) • Powders, pastes • Oil wells • Body wraps, facials
Time required	Generally a minimum of 15 days, up to 90 days	5 – 11 days	1 hour to several days

Chapter 2: Planning the Stages of Virechana

Planning for any type of Virechana or medical Pañcha Karma generally requires several months of research, education and a consistent, personal practice of Āyurveda at home. This helps to prepare you physically and mentally, reduces risks of complications, and supports you in difficult periods so that you can appreciate the process and receive the correct, long-term, beneficial outcomes.

During the research and education stage, expect to learn and practice Āyurveda on yourself for several weeks to months. This allows you to understand the principles and experience how they work in your body and mind. When adopting Āyurveda scientifically into daily life, it is common for latent sickness to rise up and cycle through. In some cases, individuals may experience sickness, fever or other general illness which may indicate that the body's immune system is activating.

As baseline physiology normalizes and strengthens, it is able to correct metabolic errors and clear out latent waste. This process often produces temporary periods of sickness while the immune system engages, repairs and restores normal health and function.

Virechana intentionally induces a state of controlled sickness in the body and often produces physical and psychological discomfort. When performed correctly, the effects produced in each stage interrupt pathological processes, halt them and reverse them. Proper Virechana can be uncomfortable and it requires continuous attention, supervision and self-discipline.

The main considerations when planning for Virechana are ultimately time and prioritization. During any form of Virechana, it is imperative to rest, minimize activities, maintain an early sleep and wake schedule, and limit meals and foods. If you are unable to commit to these requirements, do not perform Virechana. Instead, wait until you can make the time and prioritize each step of the process.

Requirements for time, space and compliance

Complete Virechana generally requires a significant time commitment of 13 to 20+ consecutive days with very limited diet and activities. Attempting to shortcut this process does not allow the deep, beneficial effects to occur, and instead will invite complications. This is ideally performed at an Āyurvedic medical facility, but can also be done at home under supervision, on a case-by-case basis.

Mini Virechana only requires 5 to 11 days and has fewer limitations on diet and activities. During the first few days of preparation, it is possible to do moderate amounts of work as long as it is not physically or mentally exhausting.

During any Virechana, prepare to have days with no planned activities. Stay in your room or space, minimize responsibilities, and expect to spend much of your time alone. Short interactions with supportive friends and family are permitted in the afternoon only. This can be an excellent opportunity for contemplative reflection, easy and enjoyable study, movies, leisure reading, arts and crafts and similar hobbies.

An ideal space has moderate, soft, natural lighting and a comfortable, warm temperature without any breeze. Quiet, dark spaces may be preferrable especially during periods of emotional instability. Throughout the procedure, avoid exposure to the external environment and elements of excess cold, heat and wind. Remain in a comfortable, climate-controlled space for the entire Virechana.

References from classical Āyurvedic literature liken the purification of Pañcha Karma and subsequent regeneration of Rasāyana to the process of dying cloth. First, the cloth must be as clean as possible so that it can fully absorb the color of the dye. A dirty cloth will not produce an even, brilliant color. Likewise, a clean body will be capable of absorbing and assimilating regenerative formulations much more effectively. To ensure high quality outcomes with purification of Pañcha Karma, these restrictions of controlled environment, avoidance of exposure to elements, timing and others are provided.

Generally, an Āyurvedic medical facility is best for Complete Virechana. Facilities usually offer a private bedroom and bathroom with hot water and access to a kitchen, or freshly prepared, appropriate meals.

Hotel or motel lodging should be avoided unless equipped with basic cooking facilities. If needed, request hypo-allergenic towels, sheets and cleaning since common detergents, disinfectants, air fresheners and other synthetic-based chemical products can be particularly irritating during Virechana.

If you choose to stay at a residential facility, expect your space to be ready when you arrive. Set up your room so that all of your clothes, personal care supplies and other necessities are organized and easily accessible. Check that your bed is comfortable and you feel content in the space.

Typically, while staying at an Āyurvedic medical facility, all your procedure and treatment supplies will be included by the facility. These generally include food, hot water, Āyurvedic medicines, oils, linens and towels, shampoo, soap, and anything else needed for the procedures. If you anticipate needing anything in particular during your stay, plan to bring it with you.

Remember that everything used during Virechana is likely to get at least a little oily. Choose simple, cotton fabrics that are breathable, and be prepared for them to become oily and potentially stained.

Treatments at an Āyurvedic medical facility should only be performed by same-sex therapists in private, usually locked, treatment rooms that have an attached bathroom. Almost all garments except underwear will need to be removed during the treatment.

Most of your time will be spent resting during the day, but not sleeping. You will need a few activities to occupy your time during the two-week procedure. Light reading, looking out the window, watching scenes of nature, looking at pictures, watching limited pleasant television, and listening to soothing music are some of the best options for passing the time. Computer and smartphone usage should be restricted for the duration of the procedure. Spending time with friends, family and loved ones will feel good in short intervals of 30 minutes or less.

Gentle physical activity like walking, stretching, Tai Chi or easy Yoga Āsana practice is usually permitted during Virechana.

Easy, organization projects can be good for this time. These things should be stress-free, like reviewing and organizing pictures, sentimental keepsakes, or other small, light and easy-to-handle items. Do not attempt anything that requires physical effort that raises your heart rate.

Simple arts and crafts projects can also be great ways to pass the time. Drawing, coloring, painting and other forms of self-expression and emotional-expression are excellent for supporting Virechana. If you are interested in spending some time on these types of activities, be sure to collect all the supplies and materials in advance and set aside a space for yourself during the process.

Finally, compliance is a major requirement for successful outcomes in Virechana. There are many rules and limitations in diet, activities, schedule, behavior, exposure to natural elements, and other details that are critical to reducing risks of complications. You must be able to follow directions and maintain self-discipline throughout the process, especially when it is difficult. If this might be challenging for you, be sure to discuss these details with your Āyurveda Āchārya during the screening process.

<table>
<tr><th>Considerations for Virechana</th><th>Complete Virechana is best</th><th>Mini Virechana is best</th></tr>
<tr><td>Time constraints</td><td>Have sufficient time, at least 14 days with no commitments</td><td>Have limited time, only a few days, may have some work that is not taxing</td></tr>
<tr><td>Space constraints</td><td>Have private, comfortable space with kitchen
OR, can stay at a facility for at least 14 days (longer for international travel)</td><td>Have private, comfortable space at home with kitchen
OR, can stay at a temporary space locally</td></tr>
<tr><td>Unable to maintain self-discipline</td><td colspan="2" rowspan="2">Facility only
OR practice Āyurveda at home under supervision until ready</td></tr>
<tr><td>Unable to remember and follow instructions</td></tr>
</table>

Screening

During the screening stage, an Āyurveda Āchārya will complete a thorough assessment of your health and medical history. Generally, this requires that you complete detailed intake forms and share relevant medical history and reports. Then, expect to meet with your Āyurveda Āchārya for about an hour. During this session, you can discuss your personal goals, and any physical and psychological issues.

At a minimum, expect to review the following personal details with your Āyurveda Āchārya.

- Your goals, understanding and expectations of Virechana
- Your medical history
    - Any diseases, symptoms and illnesses
    - Familial history
    - Use of medications (prescriptions and other drugs)
- Surgical history
- Psychological history
- Physical or psychological trauma
- For women
    - Reproductive history
    - Menstrual cycle (for planning procedures and dates)

Your Āyurveda Āchārya will explain which procedures are best for you and how to plan for them. The final determination to do any Pañcha Karma, including Virechana, will always be made collaboratively by you and your Āyurveda Āchārya.

If Virechana is not appropriate at the time of screening but you still want to experience it, your Āyurveda Āchārya may be able to work with you to create a plan of action for an extended preparation period. After several months of targeted preparation, your body and mind will likely be better prepared.

Once the determination has been made by you and your Āyurveda Āchārya that Virechana is right for you, the preparation begins. Completing the full procedure requires significant time commitments, dedication and compliance to specific, restricted routines for several weeks.

Part of this commitment includes accepting that the plan may change or require adjustments depending on how your body responds during various stages of the procedure. If this is necessary, your Āyurveda Āchārya will explain the reasons for the adjustments and ask for your compliance with changes.

Your plan for Virechana

For anyone new to Āyurveda, planning for Complete or Mini Virechana generally takes at least one week, and often much longer. The main factors that will determine your plan and schedule are based on where you intend to perform Virechana, which option you will perform (Complete or Mini), the availability of Āyurvedic medicines and other required supplies, and your confirmation of instructions, expectations and requirements.

For women in their reproductive age, Virechana must be scheduled around the menstrual cycle. Ideally, the process starts as soon as active bleeding ends. This allows the maximum amount of time for the entire procedure before the next cycle. Most importantly, the Elimination stage should be avoided with active bleeding. For some women, Stage 2: Lubrication of Complete Virechana can reset the hormonal cycle and initiate a sudden, unexpected bleeding phase. If this happens, your Āyurveda Āchārya will explain options and make a recommendation to continue or pause the procedure during the menstrual cycle. Expect to discuss your menstrual cycle in detail with your Āyurveda Āchārya during screening.

Each day throughout the entire Virechana, expect to be in touch with your Āyurveda Āchārya or Svastha Āchārya. Regular communication is key to monitoring your progress and guiding the entire procedure to a positive, successful outcome. For either form of Virechana at home, this communication replicates the attention that an in-patient or residential facility can provide for monitoring progress, outcomes and any signs of potential complications.

Depending on the mode of communication with your care team, you may be required to submit detailed information of your daily diet and activities via electronic systems. This allows your care team to monitor your progress in real time and provide better support. Additionally, expect to spend at least 15 minutes each day in contact by email, video or audio call, and up to 2 hours a day in some cases, or on certain days.

If you're unsure of what to document or discuss, include more information wherever possible. It's better to mention things which may or may not be significant than to miss one important thing. You should always feel comfortable discussing any personal health details confidentially with your Āyurveda Āchārya and Svastha Āchārya.

If you're not using an electronic record system, be sure to keep your journal and records up-to-date every day. This information can be used at any point throughout the procedure to review progress and identify issues. It is important to include as much detail as possible in your daily journal as it can help provide answers to questions later on.

Your care team	What to expect
Āyurveda Āchārya (Āyurvedic Doctor)	• Personalized, detailed assessment • Virechana plan, protocols, formulations and management • Post-protocol management
Svastha Āchārya (Āyurvedic Health Coach)	• Guidance on diet, lifestyle and activities • Instructions on meal prep, timing and methods • Training on self-observation skills • Explaining how to understand the process

Your Āyurveda Āchārya (Āyurvedic Doctor) will provide an initial overview of your specific plan. As you go through the Virechana, specific customizations and instructions may be updated day-to-day depending on how your body responds during the procedure. For any Virechana performed at home, you must be capable of keeping up with changing instructions and implementing them correctly.

Use the planning tools in the Appendix to help you plan for Mini Virechana or Complete Virechana.

Chapter 3: Compliance and Restrictions

To achieve successful outcomes in Virechana and avoid complications, there are many restrictions and few permitted activities. It is absolutely crucial that these be followed during the entire process, especially if you choose to perform any form of Virechana at home.

During various stages of the process, the body often undergoes significant changes from what would typically be considered its normal state. The following permitted activities and restrictions support these changes so that Virechana can work properly.

Often times the permitted activities and restrictions may not "feel right," and this is normal. Keep in mind that even if you don't feel like adhering to these rules, you must do so throughout the entire course of Virechana. Otherwise, serious side effects, complications or medical emergencies can occur.

The guidelines listed in this chapter are meant to be followed for the entire duration of Virechana, unless otherwise noted. Any additional guidelines for specific procedures or stages will be highlighted in later chapters or identified by your Āyurveda Āchārya. Be sure to note down any instructions that are specific to your situation. Use the tables and checklists provided in the Appendices.

Why it's so important

These guidelines help prevent mobilized waste materials (the *doṣhas*) from establishing new disease focal points as they are detached from their locations in the body. Many of these guidelines are opposite to the ways most people normally live and it can be quite easy to forget them.

This is an important reason why doing Virechana in an Āyurvedic medical facility is the safest option. It is helpful to be in a different space, away from your normal routine and lifestyle, and under constant supervision. If you find it challenging to adhere to any of these guidelines during your Virechana, you must let your Āyurveda Āchārya know in advance. You should also record it in your journal whenever possible, as it can help resolve questions later in the process.

In general, avoid anything which causes discomfort, harm, stress or exertion even at a minimal level. Consider your Virechana time to be a stress-free, activity-free staycation and an opportunity to completely slow down and rest.

What you can do

What you can do	**Why?**
Maintain regularity	Stick to the schedule and plan even if you don't understand why. Ask questions if needed.
Stay warm	Stay warm, to the point of sweating, by wearing multiple layers and using blankets whenever required. This promotes complete digestion and prevents vasoconstriction.
Stay inside	Staying inside maintains your body in a consistent environment and reduces risk of complications due to exposure to the elements. Always check with your Āyurveda Āchārya before going outside during Complete Pañcha Karma.
Use warm water	When washing any part of the body, always use warm water at or around body temperature to prevent sudden changes.
Drink hot water	All consumed water should be freshly boiled, and at or slightly above body temperature to promote digestion and metabolism.
Eat only when hungry	Only eat when feeling noticeable, continuous signs of hunger. Wait at least 4 hours after the previous meal.

What you can do	Why?
No stress	Keep your stress levels at zero, or as low as possible to prevent interfering with digestion and metabolism.
Conserve your energy	Do not exert yourself physically or mentally to conserve your energy for internal physiological activities of elimination and repair.
Release natural urges of the body	Allow all natural urges and reflexes to happen when they manifest (the urge to pass gas, urinate, move the bowels, cry, yawn, sneeze, breathe deeply, etc).
Deep, belly breathing	Perfuse the body with deep breathing to improve circulation with minimal physical activity.
Relax the muscles	Relax and soften the muscles of the body, especially in the abdomen, to promote unimpeded circulation.
Sit or stand straight	Improve posture and alignment of the entire body to allow circulation to reach areas that may have been compressed for long periods of time.
Use clothes, towels and linens of natural fibers	Wear natural fiber clothing with long sleeves that help maintain a consistent ambient environment around the body. Use socks, slippers, a hat, scarf or anything else that is needed to maintain a warm and almost sweating body temperature.

What you can't do

What you CAN'T do	Why?
Feel cold	The subjective perception of cold causes the body's vascular system to constrict which reduces circulation and perfusion. Always wear as many layers of clothing or blankets as needed to stay warm, to the point of sweating.
Doze off	Feeling tired, especially during the day, causes the digestive system to essentially turn off. This can create major complications in the procedure. Get up and walk around slowly or do something to wake up.
Eat or drink anything outside of what's permitted	The restricted diet is required to minimize indigestion which can cause severe complications.
Use any supplements or medicines	By the time you start Virechana, you should have weaned off all supplements, vitamins, minerals and other medications. These can interfere with, inhibit or mask necessary physiological changes.
Stay awake at night	Sleeping at night is a key component to establishing normal, healthy circadian rhythm and hormonal activities which cascade throughout bodily systems. Lack of sleep, difficulty sleeping or any sleep disturbance should be reported to your Āyurveda Āchārya.

What you CAN'T do	**Why?**
Overexert yourself	Do not over exert yourself physically or mentally at any point during Virechana. It can be difficult to know when to stop with activities that would normally be easily tolerated, so take a preventative approach and limit your interaction with others.
Talk too much	Same as above; limit interaction time to 30 minutes or less. Talk slowly, breathe easily and do not allow yourself to get excited.
Physical exercise	Any physical exercise that increases heart rate must be avoided to prevent sudden complications and conserve energy.
Sexual intercourse	Same as above
Stimulate the senses or use the senses incorrectly	Avoid excessive stimulation of the sense organs such as loud music, bright lights, heat, cold, dryness, dampness, etc. Avoid underuse and misuse of all sense organs.
Expose yourself to direct sunlight	Do not expose yourself to direct sunlight because the skin can be unusually sensitive during the entire procedure.
Expose yourself to direct breeze or wind	Do not expose yourself to any direct breeze or wind to avoid sensory stimulation and temperature change that can produce sudden constriction or dilation of the vascular system.

What you CAN'T do	Why?
Sudden temperature changes	Maintain your ambient environment at a stable temperature and humidity throughout the procedure to minimize complications to the vascular system.
Go outside	Same as above
Restrict natural urges	Do not withhold natural urges of the body, especially during this time. Always release them easily and appropriately.
Force natural urges	Do not force urges as this can cause unnecessary pressure on local circulation and vasculature.
Muscular tension	Do not maintain tension of the muscles because it causes obstruction of the channels in that area.
Shallow breathing	Instead, practice deep, belly breathing to improve circulation.
Improper posture	Maintain proper alignment and posture to promote proper circulation.
Personal care products	Do not use conditioner, lotion, makeup, scents, deodorant or any other personal care products after showering.

What to watch for

Throughout the entire Virechana, there are important signs and symptoms to watch for that indicate how the process is working. Many of these indicate corrections that the body is making in real-time and these signs act as important indicators in the progression of the overall procedure. Usually, the worst symptoms are experienced during the Lubrication and Elimination stages of Virechana. These begin to fade after the Recovery stage.

Remember that one of the goals of Stage 2: Lubrication of Complete Virechana, is to induce a controlled state of sickness. These signs and symptoms will result in feeling sick and cannot be suppressed.

The following list of signs and symptoms are important to monitor and record in your daily journal. Some of these signs, like nausea, gas, changes in bowel habits, or changes in appetite, are completely normal especially during Complete Virechana and should not be cause for concern.

When recording your observations, try to be as descriptive as possible, and include times, severity level and detailed descriptions wherever possible. Plan to review your observations with your Āyurveda Āchārya on a daily basis. Your observations and discussions are key to a successful outcome.

In the event of any severe signs or symptoms during any stage, contact your Āyurveda Āchārya or Svastha Āchārya immediately.

In the event of a medical emergency, call 911 or your local number for emergency responders.

What to watch for	
Common, normal	**Abnormal, requires immediate attention**
Digestive changes, mild diarrhea or constipation	Excessive diarrhea or constipation
Burps, nausea	Vomiting
Bloating, gas	Fever, extreme burning sensation
Abdominal discomfort, heat or burning	Extreme itching
Body aches, soreness, mild pain	Severe difficulty breathing
General discomfort, feeling unwell	Extreme pain, discomfort
Tingling or numbness	Loud ringing in the ears
Temporary headaches, dizziness, light-headedness, vertigo	Severe, ongoing headaches, vertigo, fainting
Discomfort when urinating	Excessive difficulty urinating, pain, slowness
Temporary increase in phlegm	Excessive phlegm (runny nose, watery eyes, mucus in the throat)
Increased or decreased waste products	Unexpected bleeding
Tiredness, exhaustion, fatigue	Severe insomnia
Temporary mood changes, emotional swings	Sudden change in sense organs or mental state

Chapter 4: Mini Virechana

Mini Virechana is the most accessible, effective and safest Mini Pañcha Karma that can be performed at home under proper supervision. The name "Mini Virechana" is a loose translation of the Āyurvedic medical phrase *Sadyo Virechana* (pronounced "sud-YO vih-RAY-chuh-nuh").

Sadyo Virechana is a Sanskrit phrase that indicates immediate or sudden elimination. It is a classical procedure in clinical practice of Āyurvedic medicine that must be performed under supervision of a qualified Āyurveda Āchārya (Āyurvedic Doctor).

The purpose of Mini Virechana is to eliminate free *pitta doṣha* which is present as various forms of metabolic waste in the body, especially in the circulatory system and liver. Only that *doṣha* which is ready to move can be eliminated with this procedure. Additional *doṣha* that is likely deeper in the system will not be affected by Mini Virechana, but may be amenable to more advanced Pañcha Karma procedures, particularly Complete Virechana.

The Mini Virechana protocol occurs in three stages, and typically requires 5 to 11 days. During the entire protocol period, many restrictions in diet, lifestyle, schedule, routine and activities must be followed to prevent complications and promote correct, positive outcomes.

Stage	**Time**	**General protocols and procedures**
Stage 1 Preparation	1 to 5 days	Specific, restricted diet Treatments like *abhyaṅga*, where indicated
Stage 2 Elimination	1 day (rarely, 2 days)	Elimination day, rest Highly restricted diet
Stage 3 Recovery	3 to 5 days	Highly restricted, gradually increasing diet to reset core digestion Rest, gradually increasing activities

Mini Virechana is generally safe to perform at home under supervision of a qualified Āyurveda Āchārya (Āyurvedic Doctor) who will screen for indications and contraindications and determine the appropriate plan, timing and methodology. Women should plan to start the process of Mini Virechana at the end of active bleeding of the menstrual cycle. This is the ideal timing, but it can also be done at other times, as instructed by the Āyurveda Āchārya.

In addition to the general rules that apply to everyone who undergoes this protocol, there are customizations that the Āyurveda Āchārya (Āyurvedic Doctor) will determine on a case-by-case basis.

Requirements and restrictions

The goal of this protocol is to reduce the total load of free *pitta doṣha*, creating an opportunity for digestive and metabolic processes to perform quick, superficial repair. In order for the body to be able to accomplish this, the following requirements and restrictions must be followed throughout the entire period.

In many cases, the initial stage of preparation may extend for several weeks prior including these requirements and restrictions. Discuss these in detail with your Svastha Āchārya so that you fully understand all of the requirements and duration of compliance.

These requirements and restrictions are the highlights from the previous chapter. Be sure to review all of the instructions in that chapter, in addition to the ones listed here.

What you **CAN** do	What you should do
Maintain a regular sleep schedule	• Go to bed around 9pm. • Be asleep by 10pm. • Wake up naturally (without an alarm) between 4 to 6am. • Get out of bed within 10 minutes.
Maintain a regular meal schedule	• Have 2, 3 or 4 meals per day. • Use whole food ingredients only. • Eat meals that include simple combinations of food, cooked properly on a stove. • Follow the specific meal and recipe instructions provided.
Drink only freshly boiled fluids	• Freshly boiled hot water • Ginger tea • Ginger and coriander tea • Or other tea as instructed
Respect your limits	• Stay within your physical and mental limits. • Do not overexert yourself. • Rest whenever needed.
Appropriate exercise and activities	• Practice correct amounts of appropriate physical exercise, as instructed.

What you **CAN'T** do	What you should NOT do
Indulge in inappropriate behavior and activities	• Do not participate in any risky behavior. • Do not put yourself in any questionable situation. • Do not participate in adventurous, high-energy or thrill-seeking activities.
Overexert yourself	• Do not overexert yourself for any amount of time physically, mentally or emotionally.
Consume excessive food or drinks	• Do not eat more than you need at any meal. • Do not snack in between meals. Wait at least 4 hours before your next meal. • Do not drink too much all at once.
Overuse, underuse or misuse your senses	• Do not expose yourself to excessive sensory stimulation via sight, hearing, smell, taste or touch. • Do not underuse any of the senses. • Do not misuse any of the senses.

What to expect afterwards

Mini Virechana allows physical waste products present in the gastrointestinal tract to be eliminated via the downward route, or rectal passage through bowel movements. This reduction of wastes also promotes a gentle reset of digestive and metabolic pathways that should be supported with an ongoing, appropriate diet and lifestyle activities.

After this procedure, it is natural to experience strong cravings for the things which contribute to dysfunction and disease. These cravings are a representation of any developing pathology attempting to continue developing by pushing the individual to indulge in disease-promoting foods and habits. This is very common, and very subversive. Most people will not even realize that they're reverting and they can quickly lose their gains.

To prepare for this, your Āyurveda Āchārya will recommend a personalized health management plan for one to three months following Mini Virechana. At a minimum, this should include:

- Ongoing follow-ups for 1 to 3 months
- Specific diet and lifestyle activities to use or avoid
- Optional use of Āyurvedic medicines to further correct underlying dysfunction
- Sattva training

Sattva training is a systematic approach for brain retraining to observe thoughts and beliefs that are likely contributing to ongoing chronic issues by creating obstructions in overall progress. This allows you to review thought patterns that are detrimental to overall, positive progress. It is a combination of approaches from current practices in Western psychology and neuroscience, based on the fundamental principles of Āyurveda and Vedic sciences.

Traditionally in India, Āyurvedic Doctors handle management very differently. They do not tell patients the names of medicines, explain treatments, or provide many details about the process. This forces the patient to completely relinquish control and trust in the doctor and practice. This component is missing outside of India and many traditional cultures, creating an obstacle in the psychological component of the healing process.

The ultimate goal is to help you achieve the best state of health possible. To reach that, dysfunction on the physical, psychological and spiritual levels must be addressed in a complete, holistic approach. This is often a long process that spans months or years, highlighted with ups and downs. Feelings of discomfort and aversion are common, and must be overcome in order to produce long-term, sustainable changes.

Sattva Training helps you to recognize, identify and disconnect inhibiting thought patterns and replace them with health-promoting thoughts. New thoughts can be anything that you are ready for, and through this process you learn how to recognize what those might be and how to amplify them.

Your care team and plan

Throughout Mini Virechana, expect to work with a team of trained and experienced healthcare professionals. Expect to be in daily contact with at least one professional via email, voice or video call.

The entire procedure is overseen and directed by your Āyurveda Āchārya (Āyurvedic Doctor). For detailed instructions on diet, lifestyle and activities, expect to work with your Svastha Āchārya (Āyurvedic Health Coach). It's best to always email both with any questions or concerns throughout the entire procedure.

Your care team	**What to expect**
Āyurveda Āchārya Āyurvedic Doctor	• Personalized assessment • Mini Virechana plan, protocols, medicines, management • Continuous monitoring with necessary adjustments • Post-protocol management
Svastha Āchārya Āyurvedic Health Coach	• Specific instructions on diet, lifestyle and activities • Explanations for meal prep, timing and methods • Training on self-observation, signs and symptoms • Explanations about the process and expectations

Work with your Āyurveda Āchārya and Svastha Āchārya to create a plan that is realistic for you. If at any time, you realize you cannot commit to something, it is your responsibility to notify your care team and work together to determine appropriate adjustments.

Your plan should include

1. Expected schedule with dates and any necessary times
2. Required materials and ingredients for the entire procedure
3. Required formulations, or Āyurvedic medicines for the entire procedure

Use the planning tools in the Appendices to create your schedule and confirm that you have all required items prior to starting. Your Āyurveda Āchārya (Āyurvedic Doctor) will instruct you on which formulations you will need and how to order them. All materials, supplies, foods and formulations must be on hand prior to starting.

Note that these items are specific for your Mini Virechana. They should not be used by anyone else without supervision from a qualified Āyurveda Āchārya. All items will not be used simultaneously, so wait for specific instructions or ask before starting anything. Extra items are included proactively in case of unexpected outcomes or complications.

If you already have any of these items on hand, confirm that they can be used. Email your Svastha Āchārya with names and photos if required. If you need to order any items, ask your Āyurveda Āchārya or Svastha Āchārya for recommendations.

Additionally, it is highly recommended to use a bidet during this process, especially for Stage 2: Elimination. If you do not have a bidet, get a portable bidet water bottle. After each bout of elimination, use the bidet to clean the area well. Then use toilet paper to dry.

Stage 1: Preparation

The goal of Stage 1 is to prepare the core digestion and metabolism located in the gastrointestinal tract so that it can process the formulations correctly in Stage 2: Elimination. In cases of chronic illness, it may take longer to complete this initial stage of preparation.

If this stage is performed incorrectly, side effects can occur later in the procedure. To determine whether core digestion is ready to move to the next stage, you can perform self-assessments several times each day. Use the digestion assessment tool in the Appendix to record your self-assessment and provide the results to your Āyurveda Āchārya.

To complete Stage 1: Preparation, use the following instructions each day. Depending on how your body responds to these steps, your Āyurveda Āchārya will determine when you are ready to move on to Stage 2: Elimination. Do not proceed to Stage 2 until your Āyurveda Āchārya confirms that you are ready.

General rules

1. Stop all formulations (internal and external) unless otherwise specified. Reduce or stop as many supplements as possible. Continue taking any prescription medications as directed by your Medical doctor, and inform your Āyurveda Āchārya and Svastha Āchārya.
2. Email at the end of each day with a detailed update including how you are feeling and if anything important or unusual happened. Your Āyurveda Āchārya will let you know if you should continue preparation or move to the next stage.
3. If you experience any signs or symptoms that are unusual or concerning, notify your Āyurveda Āchārya (Āyurvedic Doctor) and Svastha Āchārya (Āyurvedic Health Coach) by email.
4. Be prepared for a medical emergency. Know the correct numbers to call for medical help immediately. Have a plan ready knowing where you can visit an emergency room. Have any insurance or medical documentation ready.

Environment and space

1. Maintain a clean, warm space that is not too humid or too dry.

2. Protect yourself from natural elements. If you have to be outside in uncomfortable weather, make sure to dress appropriately at all times. Excessive exposure to heat, cold, wind, dampness or dryness can interrupt this process and delay the next stage.
3. Do not be exposed to wind or breeze (like a fan, or a heating or cooling vent) blowing directly on you. If your skin feels cold anywhere, cover it with more layers or blankets. You can use a heating blanket or hot water bottle for short periods (30 - 60 minutes or less).

Daily routine

1. Schedule and sleep
    a. Go to bed early. Be in bed by 9pm and asleep by 10pm.
    b. Allow yourself to wake up naturally, without an alarm.
    c. If you wake up within one hour of sunrise, get up and get out of bed within 10 minutes. Do not go back to sleep.
    d. Do not fall asleep or nap at all during the day.
    e. If you need to rest, sit in a semi-reclined position and relax for up to 45 minutes. Cover yourself with blankets and make sure you stay warm.
2. Waste and elimination
    a. Sweat often increases little by little each day. Avoid using antiperspirant and deodorant during this process.
    b. Urinary output may fluctuate in volume, flow and timing.
    c. Bowel movements may vary from loose to harder or drier, or skip a day. Fluctuations are normal and will continue through the subsequent stages.
    d. Occasionally, bowel movements may increase, or become explosive. Usually this is related to specific food or combination of foods that produces a reaction during this

stage. If this happens, be sure to record it in your journal and let your Āyurveda Āchārya (Āyurvedic Doctor) know.

e. If any of these seem unusual, notify your Āyurveda Āchārya (Āyurvedic Doctor) and Svastha Āchārya (Āyurvedic Health Coach) by email.

3. Wake up routine
   a. Immediately after waking, go to the bathroom to empty the bladder and bowels. Even if you do not notice an urge, sit on the toilet and relax. Give the body a few minutes to see if it will release any wastes as urine, gas or feces. Encourage this daily habit to promote a healthy digestive system.
   b. Using warm water only, wash your hands, rinse your face, and rinse your mouth.
   c. Brush your teeth and rinse the mouth several times with warm water. Do not use any oral rinses or mouth fresheners. Do not perform oil pulling.
   d. Drink 1 - 2 cups of freshly boiled hot water. Do not mix any cold water into the freshly boiled hot water. Just pour small amounts and let the water cool down on its own. This may promote a bowel movement, which should be passed as soon as the urge is present.
   e. Next, do a self-massage (*abhyaṅga*) for 10 - 45 minutes with plain oil (olive, coconut or sesame) or compounded oil as instructed. Apply the oil generously from head-to-toe and massage continuously over the entire body.
   f. Optionally, you may use a steam tent for 10 - 20 minutes, if instructed.
   g. Take a comfortably warm shower. Do not use very hot water that causes a sensory reaction like chills or goosebumps. Use cooler water on the head with a temperature that feels comfortable and not excessively cold.
   h. To wash the oil out of the hair and scalp, allow warm water (not hot water) to penetrate the hair completely for several minutes so that the scalp feels slightly warm and soft.

Then gently rub enough shampoo focusing on the scalp (not the hair) to create a thick lather. You can leave the shampoo in for a few minutes, or rinse immediately with warm to cool water.

   i. To wash the body, rub mild soap over the entire body with your hands, a face cloth, or a gentle brush. Avoid damaging the skin with anything too coarse or rough.
   j. Rinse off thoroughly.
   k. Get out of the shower, dry completely and get dressed while still warm.
   l. Do not apply any lotions, creams or other products unless instructed.
   m. Avoid showering or bathing at other times. If you must shower later in the day, only do it before dinner, after lunch has completely digested. Do not shower or bathe within 3 hours of eating.

4. Activities
   a. You can do low impact activities like walking or Yoga Āsana in a warm space without any wind or direct breeze. If you feel tired or unwell, avoid activities, rest and stay warm.
   b. Do not do any exercise or physical activity that feels excessive.
   c. Do not overexert or strain yourself in any way, physically, mentally or emotionally.
5. Dressing and clothing
   a. Dress appropriately. Cover the arms and legs with long sleeves at all times.
   b. Stay warm enough for the entire day so that you are almost at the point of sweating. This is a good sign that digestion and metabolism are regulating towards their normal, healthy baseline state.
   c. Watch for signs like minor shivering, feelings of anxiety or cool extremities (hands, feet, nose, cheeks, ears, etc). Any of these can indicate that you need to cover up, add more layers and stay warmer.

d. If needed, use blankets, shawls or additional layers like two pairs of pants, socks, hats, scarves, etc.

Food and fluids

1. Observation
    a. Continuously monitor and observe the body's cues for hunger and thirst.
    b. It is best to eat when hungry.
    c. Consume a total of about 8 cups (2 liters) of fluid throughout the day. This includes soup in the congee, so total water intake can be lower around 6 cups (1.5 liters) especially for individuals who tend to carry fluid easily.
2. Schedule
    a. Follow your recommended meal schedule.
    b. The ideal meal schedule is two or three meals per day.
        i. Breakfast 8a - 9a (if hungry)
        ii. Lunch 11a - 12p
        iii. Dinner 4p - 6p
    c. If you cannot sleep because you are hungry, you may need to have an additional small meal later in the evening, around 7p - 8p.
3. Consumption rules
    a. Cook what you are going to use for that day only.
    b. Do not save any cooked food to be used the next day. Leftovers can only be used if the food has been cooked 6-8 hours prior on the same day.
    c. For fluids, use a cup or container that allows you to approximately measure your total daily intake.

d. For congee meals, use the same bowl and measure your portion sizes so you know how much you are eating.
e. Monitor how much you are eating at each meal and note the amounts in your tracker.

4. Fluids
    a. All water consumed must be freshly boiled, and hot. Use an electric kettle to easily and quickly heat water when you want to drink it. Do not add cold water to cool it down.
    b. Do not force yourself to drink too much water all at once, especially with a meal.
    c. Sip on freshly boiled hot water throughout the day, and drink it in larger quantities away from meals.
    d. If too much heat feels uncomfortable, let the water cool to around body temperature, or slightly lower. Drink the water at room temperature or higher.
    e. Only use recommended herbal tea or drinks. If you notice any feelings of indigestion or sluggish digestion, drink a cup of hot ginger tea.
5. Food
    a. The ideal meal type for Stage 1: Preparation is usually congee. It may be plain, or with additional ingredients like vegetables, moong dal or chicken. Clear soups and stews can also be appropriate for this stage.
    b. Follow your personalized congee recipes and any specific recommendations.
    c. The night prior to Stage 2: Elimination, drink one glass of fresh lemon water at room temperature with a very small pinch of salt.

Stage 2: Elimination

The goal of Stage 2 is to forcefully eliminate free *pitta doṣha* from the gastrointestinal tract. This requires properly functioning baseline digestion and metabolism. This stage can only be performed with confirmation from your Āyurveda Āchārya.

General rules

1. This is the longest, hardest day of the entire process. Expect to feel more tired, exhausted and weak as the day progresses.
2. Even if you are exhausted, you must adhere to the rules for the entire day.
3. Have your congee ingredients ready on the counter so it is easy to make in the afternoon.
4. Your Āyurveda Āchārya (Āyurvedic Doctor) and Svastha Āchārya (Āyurvedic Health Coach) will be monitoring your tracker throughout the day. Please enter your information as it happens.
5. If anything unusual happens, email with an update and let your Āyurveda Āchārya and Svastha Āchārya know.
6. In case of an emergency, call for medical help immediately. Do not wait for confirmation from your Āyurveda Āchārya or Svastha Āchārya.

Environment and space

1. Stay at home for the entire day in a constant temperature environment. Do not expose yourself to sudden changes of heat, cold or breeze.
2. Do not go outside without asking your Āyurveda Āchārya, unless it is an emergency.
3. If the weather outside is warm and comfortable, you can open the windows.

Morning

1. Schedule and sleep
    a. The night before, go to bed early. Be in bed by 9pm and asleep by 10pm.
    b. Allow yourself to wake up naturally, without an alarm. You can stay in bed until sunrise.
    c. Do not fall asleep or nap at all during the day.
    d. If you need to rest, sit in a semi-reclined position and relax for up to 45 minutes. Cover yourself with blankets and make sure you stay warm. Be near the bathroom at all times.

2. Wake up routine
    a. Immediately after waking, go to the bathroom to empty the bladder and bowels, if the urge is present. If you do not have a bowel movement now, that is ok.
    b. Using warm water only, wash your hands, rinse your face, and rinse your mouth.
    c. Brush your teeth. Avoid using alcohol-based oral rinses or mouth fresheners.
    d. Drink 1 - 2 cups of freshly boiled hot water. Do not add cold water but let the water cool down on its own. This may promote a bowel movement, which should be passed as soon as the urge is present.
    e. You may be able to do a self-massage (*abhyaṅga*) for 10 - 45 minutes with plain oil. Check your specific instructions.
    f. Take a comfortably warm shower. Do not use very hot water that causes a sensory reaction like chills or goosebumps. Use cooler water on the head with a temperature that feels comfortable and not excessively cold.
    g. You will shower again in the evening, without doing *abhyaṅga*.
3. Dressing and clothing
    a. Wear comfortable, breathable clothing that you can remove easily to use the bathroom.
    b. Do not wear anything tight around the waist.
4. Mini Virechana
    a. After showering, put 2 - 3 cups (about 0.5 liters) of water on to boil in the kettle.
    b. Next, you will take the formulation that will induce purgation for the day. Your Āyurveda Āchārya will give you the name of the specific formulation(s) you should use, their quantity and any special instructions on how to consume them.
    c. Use the following instructions to prepare it and consume your specific dose.
    d. If not listed here, your Āyurveda Āchārya will provide instructions separately.

Select common formulations with examples of usage instructions **Follow specific instructions provided by your Āyurveda Āchārya.**	
Avipatti chūrṇa (powder)	• Start with ½ packet, and empty it into a cup. • Add about ½ cup freshly boiled hot water and mix well. • Consume the entire amount, while hot. Drink more hot water in between if you feel uncomfortable. • Wait about 3-5 minutes, and if you feel ok, take the remaining ½ packet in the same way. • If instructed, take more in the same way.
Trivrit leham, or Trivrilleham (paste)	• Measure the specified amount on a spoon using a digital scale. • Lick the paste and let it dissolve in your mouth. • Drink freshly boiled hot water to help it go down. • Wait about 3-5 minutes, and if you feel ok, take an additional 5 grams (1 flat teaspoon). • If instructed, take more in the same way.
Triphala chūrṇa (powder)	• Bring 1.5 cups of water to boil in a small pot. Reduce heat to simmer. • Add 1 heaping tablespoon of triphala powder and stir immediately. If the heat is too high, it will bubble over quickly. • Bring the mixture to a gentle simmer for 30 to 60 seconds, then remove from heat. • Let it rest for a few minutes so the powder settles. Siphon the liquid off the top into a cup and drink ½ cup. • Wait about 3-5 minutes, and if you feel ok, consume another ½ cup. • If instructed, take more in the same way.
Gandharvahastadi tailam OR Castor oil	• Start with 1 teaspoon of oil. • Consume it directly from the spoon, or mixed in a little bit of freshly boiled hot water. Drink more hot water if needed to wash it down. • Wait about a minute, and if you feel ok, take an additional 1 teaspoon. • If instructed, take more in the same way.

5. What to expect 1-2 hours after the formulation
    a. Some formulations can produce immediate or delayed sensations of nausea, discomfort, heat, sweat, itching, headaches, dizziness and other symptoms.
    b. If you feel the urge to vomit, do not suppress it. Go to the bathroom immediately and allow it to come out easily. Afterwards, use warm water to rinse your mouth and wash your hands and face. Email for further instructions.
    c. If you do not vomit, just continue to sip on freshly boiled hot water when thirsty. Alternate between gently walking, stretching, and sitting while waiting for bowel movements to begin. Make sure to stay warm to the point of sweating, or the bowel movements may not begin. Stay bundled up in heavy clothes and blankets and apply a hot water bottle to your lower abdomen, or sit in a sunny window inside.
    d. Usually bowel movements start within 30 to 90 minutes. If they do not start, contact your Āyurveda Āchārya for instructions no later than 2 hours.

Midday (elimination period)

1. Activities
    a. Drink freshly boiled hot water (2-3 liters total). Have about ½ to 1 cup of freshly boiled hot water after each bout of elimination.
    b. Go to the bathroom as soon as you feel the urge. Sometimes it may be extremely urgent. Stay close to the bathroom all day.
    c. Use the bidet after each bowel movement to prevent unnecessary irritation to the area. Follow this with light tapping of toilet paper to dry the area.
    d. Walk around the house gently, or do very slow, easy stretches, but do not force it if you feel tired.

e. Sit in a comfortable chair, or recliner, but do not lie down. Be sure to stay completely warm for the entire day.
f. Do not overexert or strain yourself in any way, physically, mentally or emotionally.

2. Bowel movements and tracking
   a. Expect 5 - 15 bowel movements over the course of the day.
   b. Stool will initially be normal and formed.
   c. After 1-3 bouts, it will change to a soft mass and then become liquid with or without debris particles.
   d. Liquid usually starts as brown, and then may change to greenish or yellow, and finally may become clear.
   e. If you notice blood in your stool at any time email your Āyurveda Āchārya immediately.
   f. Track each of your bowel movements with time, urgency, color and consistency.
   g. Also track any burps, and notice if there is any lingering taste of the formulation. Once it is fully digested, the taste will go away.
   h. Observe and monitor your levels of fatigue, discomfort, pain and other symptoms. Note them in your tracker with the bowel movements.
   i. Around 12p - 2p you may feel extremely tired. Do not fall asleep. Get up and walk around or do something to stay awake.

Late afternoon (after elimination)

1. After bowel movements finish
   a. Between 3 - 6p you should start to feel light, hungry, tired, and that bowel movements are slowing down or stopping completely. When these signs appear, take a warm (not too hot) shower. Start preparing the congee now, so it is ready when you are hungry.

b. During and after your shower, notice if you have any burps. If you can taste the formulation, that means it has not completely digested and you cannot eat yet. Instead, continue to drink more hot water after showering and wait until the burps are clear (no taste of any formulation).

2. Initial recovery meal: hot, soupy, simple carbohydrates only
    a. Today, you will consume very little food. The core digestion and metabolism has been pushed hard, and can only tolerate very light congee soup water or thin congee.
    b. Prepare plain congee from the Appendix recipe, Recovery meal #1, Congee Water
    c. Sit quietly and comfortably and pay attention while eating.
    d. If you notice feeling full quickly, do not force any more.
    e. If you cannot eat much, or you eat early and you feel hungry again in the next 3 - 4 hours, you can have one more small serving in the same way.

Nighttime

1. Rest and sleep
    a. Rest for the remainder of the evening.
    b. Wait 60 minutes before lying down.
    c. Go to bed as early as you want.
2. Communication
    a. Record all your details in your journal or tracker by the end of the day while it is still fresh in your mind.
    b. If there is anything else you want to share, send an email with an update. This is not necessary if you have entered everything into an electronic tracker.

Stage 3: Recovery

The goal of Stage 3 is to recover and restore from the intensity of elimination day which takes a heavy toll on the body, digestion and metabolism. Everyone needs at least 3 days before they start eating their normal foods and meals in regular quantities. Be prepared to need additional days of restoration, based on how your body responds during this stage.

This stage of the entire process is the most important. It is like restarting the digestive system after a reboot. It strengthens digestion and metabolism to the best levels possible in this process.

Any of the following can interfere with recovery and potentially cause longer-term damage to the digestive system. All of the following must be avoided during this stage:

- Eating too much, according to one's feeling of fullness (not by measured food quantity)
- Eating too frequently, before the previous meal has fully digested
- Snacking
- Cold food, meals or fluids
- Incompatible food combinations
- Consuming food and/or fluids together in incompatible ways

Each day, you will follow the same routine and meal schedule. Meals will gradually increase, starting from a congee base, and then flavored with specific vegetables, flavors or spices. This entrains the core digestion and metabolism for optimal performance and function.

It is extremely important that this step be completed in its entirety, according to your specific instructions. If you find that you are extremely hungry or need to change something, email your Āyurveda Āchārya and Svastha Āchārya. Explain what is happening and what you feel you need. Remember, sudden changes in diet during this time can cause very uncomfortable side effects, long-term serious conditions, or emergencies.

General rules

1. Do not use any formulations (internal or external) or other supplements unless otherwise specified. Continue taking any medications as prescribed.
2. Email at the end of each day with a detailed update including how you feel and if anything important or unusual happened. Your Āyurveda Āchārya and Svastha Āchārya will let you know if there are any changes needed for the next day.
3. If you experience any signs or symptoms that are not described below, or that seem unusual, notify your Āyurveda Āchārya (Āyurvedic Doctor) and Svastha Āchārya (Āyurvedic Health Coach) by email.
4. In case of an emergency, call for medical help immediately.

Environment and space

1. Maintain a clean, warm space that is not too humid or too dry. You will likely feel more sensitive to cold and changes in ambient temperature.
2. Protect yourself from the natural elements as much as possible. Avoid going outside in extreme temperatures or conditions. If you have to go outside, make sure to dress appropriately at all times. Exposure to heat, cold, wind, dampness or dryness can interrupt the recovery process and hinder restoration of core digestion and metabolism.
3. Do not be exposed to wind or breeze (like a heating or cooling vent) blowing directly on you. If your skin feels cold anywhere, cover it with more layers or blankets. You can use a heating blanket or hot water bottle for short periods (30 - 60 minutes or less).

Daily routine

1. Schedule and sleep
    a. Go to bed early. Be in bed by 9pm and asleep by 10pm.

   b. Allow yourself to wake up naturally, without an alarm. Whenever you wake up after 5am, get up and get out of bed within 10 minutes. Do not go back to sleep.
   c. Do not fall asleep or nap at all during the day.
   d. If you need to rest, sit in a semi-reclined position and relax for up to 45 minutes. Cover yourself with blankets and make sure you stay warm.
2. Waste and elimination
   a. Sweat can vary during this stage, depending on the overall state of health. For generally healthy individuals, sweat may decrease slightly. For individuals with chronic disease, sweat and body odor can increase significantly. Avoid using antiperspirant and deodorant during this process.
   b. Urinary output may fluctuate in volume, flow and timing.
   c. Bowel movements will likely not happen for 2-3 days if you experienced a large amount of elimination in Stage 2.
   d. If any of these seem unusual, notify your Āyurveda Āchārya (Āyurvedic Doctor) and Svastha Āchārya (Āyurvedic Health Coach) by email.
3. Wake up routine
   a. Immediately after waking, go to the bathroom to empty the bladder and bowels, if the urge is present.
   b. Using warm water only, wash your hands, rinse your face, and rinse your mouth.
   c. Brush your teeth. Avoid using alcohol-based oral rinses or mouth fresheners.
   d. Drink 1 - 2 cups of freshly boiled hot water. Do not add cold water but let the water cool down on its own. This may promote a bowel movement, which should be passed as soon as the urge is present.
   e. If recommended for your specific situation, you may start *abhyaṅga* on the 3rd day after Stage 2.

f. Do a self-massage (*abhyaṅga*) for 10 - 45 minutes with plain oil (olive, coconut or sesame), applying oil head-to-toe, according to your specific instructions.
g. Optionally, you may use a steam tent for 10 - 20 minutes, if instructed.
h. Take a comfortably warm shower. Do not use very hot water that causes a sensory reaction like chills or goosebumps. Use cooler water on the head with a temperature that feels comfortable and not excessively cold.
i. Do not apply any lotions, creams or other products unless instructed.
j. Avoid showering or bathing at other times. If you must shower later in the day, only do it before dinner, after lunch has completely digested. Do not shower or bathe within 3 hours of eating.

4. Activities
    a. You will feel progressively better and stronger each day during recovery. Pace yourself and limit your activities according to your strength and energy levels. Do not overexert yourself and take the time to pause and rest when needed.
    b. You can do low impact activities like walking or Yoga Āsana in a warm space without any wind or direct breeze. If you feel tired or unwell, avoid activities and stay warm instead.
    c. Do not overexert or strain yourself in any way, physically, mentally or emotionally.
    d. Towards the end of this stage, you can test your limits and push yourself in activities that increase heart rate and break a sweat.
5. Dressing and clothing
    a. Dress appropriately. Cover the arms and legs with long sleeves.
    b. Stay warm enough for the entire day so that you are almost at the point of sweating. This will support recovery of digestion and metabolism.

c. Watch for signs like minor shivering, feelings of anxiety, extremities that feel cool to touch (hands, feet, nose, cheeks, ears, etc). Any of these can indicate that you need to cover up and stay warmer.
d. If needed, use blankets, shawls or additional layers like two pairs of pants, socks, etc.

Food and fluids

1. Observation
    a. Continuously monitor and observe the body's cues for hunger, thirst, digestion and output.
    b. It is best to eat when hungry. The recovery period is the ideal time to become aware of your circadian rhythms and natural hunger peaks. Plan your days around these times so that your system can function optimally.
    c. Consume a total of about 8 cups (2 liters) of fluid throughout the day. This includes soup in the congee, so total water intake may be around 6 cups (1.5 liters).
2. Schedule
    a. Follow your recommended meal schedule.
    b. The ideal meal schedule is three meals per day.
        i. Breakfast 8a - 9a (if hungry)
        ii. Lunch 11a - 12p
        iii. Dinner 4p - 6p
    c. Wait at least 3 hours before eating your next meal, if you had a small meal.
    d. Wait at least 4 - 6 hours before eating your next meal, if you had a large meal that was heavy or filling.
    e. Do not snack at all between meals. If you are extremely hungry, eat more at each meal and find the right portion size that satisfies you.

    f. If you cannot sleep because of hunger, you may need to have an additional small meal later in the evening, around 7p - 8p. Email your Āyurveda Āchārya and Svastha Āchārya to confirm.

3. Consumption rules
    a. Cook what you are going to use for that day only.
    b. Do not save any cooked food to be used the next day. Leftovers can only be used if the food has been cooked 6-8 hours prior on the same day.
    c. For fluids, use a cup or container that allows you to approximately measure your total daily intake.
    d. For congee meals, use the same bowl and measure portion sizes so you know how much you are eating, and if you are eating more or less each day.
4. Fluids
    a. All water consumed must be freshly boiled, and hot. Use a kettle to easily heat the water when you want to drink it. Do not add cold water to cool it down.
    b. Do not force yourself to drink too much water all at once, especially with meals that contain a higher proportion of liquid.
    c. Sip on freshly boiled hot water throughout the day, and drink it in larger quantities away from meals.
    d. If too much heat feels uncomfortable, let the water cool to around body temperature, or slightly lower. Drink the water at room temperature or higher.
    e. Only use recommended herbal tea.
5. Food
    a. During this stage, meals will gradually increase in density, heaviness and ingredients. Follow your specific instructions each day.

Principles of the Recovery Stage

Mini Virechana produces significant changes in the physiology and homeostasis of the gastrointestinal tract relatively quickly. Because of the sudden elimination of the contents of the digestive system, the body needs time and a simplified diet to recalibrate during the Recovery Stage. This allows the entire system, including gut microbiome, to reset itself safely, easily and effectively. Very importantly, it also helps to avoid side effects and longer-term complications.

The Recovery Stage may last several days or more, depending on the specific condition of the individual, the starting point, chronicity and other factors in the presentation. Your Āyurveda Āchārya will provide a clear plan for each day of the Recovery Stage with instructions for routine, lifestyle activities and diet. Plan to stick to these instructions for as long as required to maximize positive outcomes.

The gradual progression of the diet during the Recovery Stage allows subsequently heavier macronutrients to be reintroduced in a specific order. This reprograms the digestive system and allows it to achieve an optimal state of functioning in its current condition.

1st step	→	Liquid, carbohydrate only, plus salt
	→	Solid, carbohydrate only, plus salt
2nd step	→	Add protein
3rd step	→	Add fat
4th step	→	Regular, light, easy-to-digest meal

In Āyurvedic medicine, the principles of this sequence are based on the process of digestion in the body, starting from the tongue and saliva. Each progressive step moves deeper into the digestive tract to challenge it to function properly.

Chapter 5: Complete Virechana

Complete Virechana includes five main stages followed by a longer post-virechana period. The five main stages require a minimum of 13 days. The post-virechana period typically lasts 90 to 180 days.

Each stage is performed to achieve a specific goal towards the final outcome. It is designed to alter normal physiology to allow for the safe elimination of accumulated waste products (*doṣhas*).

Each stage also has a few main activities that are the focus for that time. Some of these activities may be done at home, while others may be performed in a facility by trained therapists under supervision of an Āyurveda Āchārya.

The Complete Virechana protocol occurs in five stages and usually requires about 14 days.

Stage	**Time**	**General protocols and procedures**
Stage 1 Preparation	3 – 7 days	• Specific, restricted diet to increase digestive capacity • Drying treatments, where indicated
Stage 2 Lubrication	3 – 7 days	• Overwhelming the gastrointestinal tract with fat (ghee or oil) to reach saturation point
Stage 3 Mobilization	3 days	• Loosening and mobilizing adhered metabolic wastes into circulation for elimination
Stage 4 Elimination	1 day (rarely 2 days)	• Elimination day, rest • Highly restricted diet
Stage 5 Recovery	3 – 7 days	• Highly restricted, gradually building diet to reset core digestion and metabolism • Rest, limited activities

The complete protocol can take anywhere from 13 to 25 days, or more in rare cases. During the entire protocol period, many restrictions in diet, lifestyle, schedule, routine and activities must be followed to prevent complications and promote positive outcomes.

Time commitment

The time commitment needed for Complete Virechana is usually one of the biggest obstacles. To ensure a successful outcome with minimal or no complications, one must have at least 13 continuous days with minimal activities, responsibilities or other commitments. Practically, this means no work, no going out of the house, no physical exercise, and very limited, short duration activities.

Stage 1 can be mostly completed at home over 3 to 30 days. It usually requires adjustments to diet and lifestyle activities to prepare the body for the rest of the procedure. Stage 1 begins once you and your Āyurveda Āchārya decide that Complete Virechana is appropriate for you. Your Āyurveda Āchārya will provide instructions on diet, lifestyle, self-care and any formulations that will support the preparation.

In some cases, more than 30 days are required to prepare. And it's possible that plans may change during the preparation period for many reasons. In these cases, Stage 1 will be extended as needed.

Stages 2 through 5 cover the main period which is best managed in a residential facility under direct supervision and continuous observation. The arrival and departure days are not included in the total time required for the procedure. These stages can be done at home in select cases with sufficient preparation and daily monitoring via online, video calls.

Post-Virechana is the regenerative period of 40 to 180 days or more following a Complete Virechana. This can be done completely at home with proper adjustments to diet and lifestyle activities. This period is the most important in changing long-term health. Habits that may have contributed to ill health are actively avoided during this time to prevent possible relapse. Āyurvedic formulations are almost always used to promote regeneration during this period.

For women in their reproductive age, Complete Virechana must be scheduled around the menstrual cycle. Ideally, Stage 2: Lubrication starts as soon as active bleeding ends. This allows the maximum amount of time for the entire procedure before the next cycle. Most importantly, the Elimination stage should be avoided with active bleeding. For some women, Stage 2: Lubrication of Complete Virechana can reset the hormonal cycle and initiate a sudden, unexpected bleeding phase. If this happens, your Āyurveda Āchārya will explain options and make a recommendation to continue or pause the procedure during the menstrual cycle. Expect to discuss your menstrual cycle in detail with your Āyurveda Āchārya during screening.

Estimate your schedule for Virechana using the guide in the Appendix. Your Āyurveda Āchārya will provide estimates for the number of days needed in each stage. Then, you can decide which dates work best and plan accordingly.

Supplies

A variety of supplies, Āyurvedic medicines and foods are typically required throughout a Complete Virechana. If staying at a residential facility during Stages 2 through 5, expect these supplies, medicines and foods to be provided.

If performing a Complete Virechana at home, you must source and obtain all required supplies prior to starting the procedure. If possible, plan to have a small number of fresh vegetables delivered about half way through the process to be used during Stage 5. See the Appendix for planning checklists.

Mindset

Due to the many restrictions that must be followed during the process, it is often too stressful to be able to complete a normal day work or activities.

The purpose of Complete Virechana is to change the body's state of health on many levels relatively quickly. In order to do that successfully, you must prioritize your physical and mental needs and create an environment that promotes rest and stress management in a healthy way.

A full, Complete Virechana is a challenging process physically, mentally and emotionally. It requires that the body and mind be allowed to rest completely for the duration of the process and possibly for several weeks afterwards, depending on the individual and specific health issues. For many people who are used to a "Go – Go – Go" type of lifestyle, resting can be one of the most challenging aspects of the entire process.

While preparing for Complete Virechana, use the time during Stage 1: Preparation to switch gears into a slower, gentler routine. Take at least a few days to allow yourself to indulge in restful activities like reading a relaxing book, watching a pleasant movie or going on a gentle stroll in a park.

Spending an hour or two like this for a few days leading up to Stage 2 will help calm the mind and stabilize it. Otherwise, a sudden change of pace from a "Go – Go – Go" routine to the "Slow – Slow – Slow" resting routine of Complete Virechana can be difficult.

During Stage 2: Lubrication, it is common for latent or hidden emotions to surface. Large quantities of fat consumption during this stage quickly interrupt and alter hormonal pathways and can lead to unpredictable emotional states. Many people find that they have sudden shifts in emotional states, feel mentally unstable, not in their "norm" and may even start crying or experience other emotional extremes for no apparent reason. This is normal and part of the internal restructuring process.

As such, strong and variable emotional states should not be taken as a major cause for concern unless they have the potential to cause harm. The best way to manage emotions as they arise during Stage 2 is to spend time on introspection, journaling and reflection while allowing emotions, thoughts and feelings to express themselves in a healthy way. It can also be very helpful to have a supportive loved one with whom you can talk things through and process emotional changes.

Often these feelings are tightly related to underlying physical imbalances and encouraging their release can significantly aid the overall success of the process. Having the support of a trusted loved one to provide comfort and guidance can be a great benefit. It is imperative that this supportive person be aware of Complete Virechana and its role in emotional instability. This helps everyone remember that it is part of the process and should be handled in a healthy, comforting way.

What to watch for

Throughout Complete Virechana, important signs and symptoms indicate how the process is working. Many of these indicate corrections that the body is making in real-time and these signs act as important indicators in the progression of the overall procedure. Usually, the most challenging or difficult symptoms are experienced during the Stage 2: Lubrication and Stage 4: Elimination. These begin to fade after Stage 5: Recovery.

Remember that one of the goals of Stage 2: Lubrication is to induce a controlled state of sickness. These signs and symptoms often result in feeling sick. While they cannot be suppressed, your Āyurveda Āchārya will likely be able to help you work through them to minimize their effect. Be sure to ask if you need help working through any physical, mental or emotional problems during the entire process.

The following list of signs and symptoms are important to monitor and record in your daily journal. Common signs like moderate nausea, gas, changes in bowel habits, or changes in appetite are completely normal especially during Complete Virechana and should not be cause for concern.

Try to be as descriptive as possible when recording your observations and include times, severity level and detailed descriptions wherever possible. Plan to review your observations with your Āyurveda Āchārya on a daily basis. Your observations and discussions are essential to a successful outcome.

In the event of any severe signs or symptoms during any stage, contact your Āyurveda Āchārya or Svastha Āchārya immediately.

In the event of a medical emergency, call 911 or your local number for emergency responders.

What to watch for	
Common, normal	**Abnormal, requires immediate attention**
Digestive changes, mild diarrhea or constipation	Excessive diarrhea or constipation
Burps, nausea	Vomiting
Bloating, gas	Fever, extreme burning sensation
Abdominal discomfort, heat or burning	Extreme itching
Body aches, soreness, mild pain	Severe difficulty breathing
General discomfort, feeling unwell	Extreme pain, discomfort
Tingling or numbness	Loud ringing in the ears
Temporary headaches, dizziness, light-headedness, vertigo	Severe, ongoing headaches, vertigo, fainting
Discomfort when urinating	Excessive difficulty urinating, pain, slowness
Temporary increase in phlegm	Excessive phlegm (runny nose, watery eyes, mucus in the throat)
Increased or decreased waste products	Unexpected bleeding
Tiredness, exhaustion, fatigue	Severe insomnia
Temporary mood changes, mood swings	Sudden change in sense organs or mental state

A typical day during Complete Virechana

Specific daily activities should be followed for the duration of Virechana, particularly Stages 2 through 5. There are also recommendations which can help make the process more comfortable and support a successful outcome.

Although it's not necessary to adhere to every recommendation during Stage 1, it is strongly advised to transition towards these activities and schedule especially if they are very different from what you're used to. Some of these activities, like waking up before sunrise, must be aligned before Stage 2 can begin. This indicates circadian rhythm is in sync and there is risk when consuming fats.

Review what a typical day looks like during Virechana. Note any activities that might be a challenge for you and start working on them early in the process. Be sure to discuss your current routine and any of these activities which may be challenging for you with your Āyurveda Āchārya.

A Typical Day during Virechana (Stages 2 through 5)		
Time	Activity	Explanation
30 to 60 min before sunrise	Wake up	Train the body to synchronize its normal circadian rhythm. This provides a healthy foundation for all internal physiology.
Immediately after waking	Personal hygiene	Go to the bathroom and empty the bladder and bowels if the urge is present. Immediately wash your hands and face with warm or tepid water, rinse the mouth, expel any phlegm or mucous from the throat and brush the teeth.
About 15-20 min before sunrise	Prepare first drink	Boil fresh water thoroughly. During Stage 2, fats will be consumed before water.
At sunrise	Consume fats (ghee or oil), followed by hot water	During Stage 2, consume your entire dose of fats for the day at sunrise. Follow the procedure detailed later in this chapter. In all other stages, sip one to two cups of freshly boiled hot water.
After sunrise	Gentle movement, stretching, breathing	During Stage 2, alternate slowly walking with sitting down to sip on hot water. In all other stages, gentle movement, stretching and breathing improves metabolism and circulation.
Around 8am	Breakfast	During Stages 3 and 5, breakfast can be included in the routine. Depending on the stage and day, it may be a flavored version of congee. This will be customized for you at that time.

Around 9am	Treatments	During Stage 3, external treatments may be performed between breakfast and lunch, or on rising.
Around 12pm	Lunch	Lunch normally consists of congee. In Stage 5 it will include light flavors. Lunch at the normal time (around noon) does not happen during some of the stages.
After lunch	Light activities to avoid falling asleep	After lunch it is important to do something light, easy and enjoyable to prevent tiredness or falling asleep. Gentle strolls, simple projects, and other non-stressful activities are good ways to stay engaged while not over-working the body.
Around 4pm	Evening snack, if necessary	For some people, congee will not be filling enough to last more than a few hours. On the days when you're consuming more meals, especially during Stage 3, an extra bowl of congee in the evening can help keep the digestive power stable. Before consuming an extra bowl at this time, ask your Āyurveda Āchārya.
Around 6-7pm	Dinner	Dinner time may be earlier or later depending on the total number of meals consumed during the day. The last meal should not be too early or it can be difficult to fall asleep.
Around 9pm or earlier	Get ready for bed	Sleep can often be difficult during Virechana. It is recommended to get into bed as soon as you feel tired, around 9pm or earlier. Try reading a very boring book or watching very quiet, boring television for just a short time if you need help falling asleep.

Stage 1, Preparation

Appetite stimulation (*dīpana*) and digestion promotion (*pāchana*)

Purpose and duration

The process of Complete Virechana begins with the preparation of the digestive system. In Āyurvedic medicine, this includes stimulating the appetite (*dīpana*) and strengthening the power of digestion to metabolize remnant wastes (*pāchana*).

Stimulation of the appetite strengthens intake capacity and increases it. Promotion of digestion improves metabolism, the ability to break down and assimilate consumed items for further processing throughout the body. These two function interdependently and their peak performance is an indicator that Stage 2: Lubrication can begin.

The methodologies used to achieve these results are generally applied using internal Āyurvedic medicines in conjunction with external, therapeutic treatments. Classical literature likens the effects of stimulating the appetite (*dīpana*) and metabolizing remnant wastes (*pāchana*) to the power of the sun (*dīpana*), and the sun and wind (*pāchana*) to dry up standing water. The sun alone can dry small puddles easily, while the sun and wind combined are more effective with larger quantities of water. In these similes, the water represents the stagnant pools of *doṣhas* (metabolic waste) in the physical body. The third component of this analogy describes the total effect of Virechana, which facilitates the removal of excess *doṣhas* from their nearest physiological route of exit. In this analogy, water breaches its dam and overflows to be released. Similarly, with Complete Virechana, the quantum of *doṣhas* in the physical body is purposefully increased so that it can overflow and be released through its nearest exit in the gastrointestinal system, either from the upward (oral) or downward (rectal) route.

To achieve a strong appetite and digestion, the body must be moderately dried internally, particularly in the gastrointestinal tract (*koṣhṭha*). This process of drying is called *rūkṣhaṇa* and it causes the physical body to become more dry, rough and light. For some, this may result in temporary symptoms like constipation, irritability, dry skin, eyes or hair, joint pain or stiffness. Presentation of symptoms during this stage is normal as the underlying pre-disease components are slightly exposed by *dīpana*, *pāchana* and *rūkṣhaṇa*.

Stage 1 is the most flexible stage of the entire process. It can be completed in as little as 3 days or require several months of sequential interventions. However, the strength of the appetite and digestion that is generated during this stage is directly responsible for the effectiveness of the rest of the entire procedure.

General recommendations

During this stage, some dietary and lifestyle recommendations may be similar to your normal routine. All meals should be hot, freshly cooked, light, easy to digest, and gently spiced. There are a variety of foods and meals that can meet these criteria including one-pot style soups and stews, simple combinations of a single grain with a single vegetable (stir fry, steamed, baked, etc), single protein source with light spices and a vegetable, etc.

A good rule to follow is to use the fewest ingredients necessary to create an enjoyable meal. The goal is to reduce the burden of confusion on the digestive system so that it can process what it's given easily and more effectively. This optimizes its activity and functioning, helps to clear various channels throughout the body, and stabilizes the mind.

During Stage 1, review your current lifestyle and routine and start aligning it towards a typical day in Virechana (described in the previous section). Most importantly, your sleep and wake times must be naturally aligned to sunrise before starting Stage 2: Lubrication.

If this is very different from your typical routine, plan to spend at least 1 to 2 weeks practicing by slowing yourself down early at night (around 8pm), getting ready for bed by 9pm, and being in bed before 9:30pm, with lights out. It is imperative that you make every attempt to fall asleep before 10pm in order to allow the digestive system time to recover, which happens approximately between 10pm and 2am.

Waking up half an hour before sunrise is equally important to align the natural circadian rhythm and support the varied systems of metabolic and endocrinal activities that depend on these internal clocks.

Wherever possible, also try to slow down your general activity levels so that it doesn't feel like a shock to sit inside and "do nothing" for two weeks. Favor exercises that allow you to focus on your body's needs and go at your own pace. Tai Chi or Yoga Āsanas are excellent when practiced independently and you can take your time to recognize any physical issues that your body might be dealing with. Be as fully aware of these issues as possible by gently pushing their limits through controlled stretching, self-massage and slow, simple weight-bearing exercises using only your body weight.

Keep a detailed list of these physical issues in your journal as important "before" signs of your current physical state. Certain issues like muscular tightness, stiffness, inflexibility and restriction of joint movement can be targeted during Complete Virechana to try to open and release them. Always mention these issues to your Āyurveda Āchārya and discuss them during the process for best management.

And whenever possible, the body and general strength levels should be built up prior to Stage 1 so that Complete Virechana doesn't end up doing more damage than good. Anyone in a lower weight category, or who generally has trouble gaining weight, will need to address this before starting Stage 1.

Regular, healthy meals and regular, appropriate exercise are key to building the body's strength and capacity. Discuss specifics with your Āyurveda Āchārya and formulate a plan together to prepare within a realistic time frame for your level of commitment and dedication.

You may also be required to perform certain types of hot, drying treatments on yourself during this stage if you're performing Complete Virechana at home to support *rūkṣhaṇa*. In a facility, expect to receive one to two treatments per day that will most likely include dry powder, pouring of warm, water-based herbal extractions, or other dry heat treatments. Oil-based treatments are almost always contraindicated during this preparatory stage.

Your dietary recommendations

Your Āyurveda Āchārya may provide additional, specific dietary recommendations for you to use during Stage 1 to prepare your digestive system more effectively. These recommendations are specific to your current state of health, the season and the intended outcome of Complete Virechana. They should be followed as directed. Be sure that you understand all preparation and cooking instructions well.

Note your specific dietary recommendations in the Stage 1: Preparation section of the Appendix.

Your lifestyle recommendations

Any specific lifestyle recommendations that will help prepare the digestive system more effectively should be listed here. Your Āyurveda Āchārya may recommend that you prioritize certain activities and those should be included in this list.

Note your specific activity recommendations in the Stage 1: Preparation section of the Appendix.

Your self-care treatments

External treatments can play a supportive role in preparing the digestive system in a variety of ways. These treatments are best done by a qualified therapist who is trained to perform them. In special situations, they can also be performed at home on yourself, however, it is almost impossible to get the same beneficial results without being able to relax during the treatment. If external treatments are supportive in your specific situation, your Āyurveda Āchārya will let you know and help you determine the best way to do them.

Note your specific self-care treatment recommendations in the Stage 1: Preparation section of the Appendix.

Āyurvedic formulations

In most cases, additional internal formulations are utilized to help prepare the digestive system effectively. These formulations are designed to focus on a specific aspect or function of the digestive power, processing ability, output or capacity and enhance it. In classical Āyurveda, dozens of formulations are available to produce these effects but their availability outside of India fluctuates. Your Āyurveda Āchārya will provide a list of recommended items that are appropriate for you and direct you on how to order them.

Note your specific formulation recommendations in the Stage 1: Preparation section of the Appendix. Review all of your formulations prior to starting Stage 2. Make sure they are shaken and ready for use.

Stage 2, Lubrication

Preparatory stage (*pūrva karma*) to excite the *doṣhas*, with internal lubrication (*abhyantara snehana*)

Overview

Every day during Stage 2: Lubrication the general procedure for heating and consuming the fat is nearly the same. The main difference is that the quantity of fat increases daily, along with its required duration for digestion. The total number of days for consuming fat is customized for each person, on a day-to-day basis.

Your Āyurveda Āchārya will outline your plan for Lubrication but depending on what actually happens and how you respond, daily adjustments may be required.

Use the planning tools in the Appendix to note instructions from your Āyurveda Āchārya. Then, record your activities, self-assessments and any results in the daily charts. Be sure to clearly write down the quantity of fat indicated for that day, along with the date at the top. Charts have been provided for seven days but you may not need to use all of them.

Purpose and duration

Stage 2: Lubrication is the phase that readies the body to expel accumulated waste products (*doṣhas*) by separating them from any structures or tissues that they are attached to in the body. The liberal use of fats is the key to achieving this goal in Stages 2 and 3.

Fats act as a surfactant and allow the minute separation of waste material from healthy bodily tissues. Simple examples can demonstrate this principle in action. If you've ever gotten your hands dirty with thick grease, you'll know that regular soap and water are not always effective at removing it. The best way to remove stubborn, stuck grease is with an oil-based surfactant. This is the role that fats play in Stages 2 and 3.

Every cell of the human body is formed by fat molecules which create a double layer, phospholipid membrane. This creates a strong wall of protection around the cell, and allows the cell to regulate transportation of other molecules and compounds across the membrane. Over time, these fats often become damaged as part of the natural aging process. The superfluous intake of fats during Stage 2 provide a large supply of new fat molecules for the body to replenish and repair internal structures. Fats can additionally cross the blood-brain barrier, and naturally have strong cohesion which likely allow them to permeate deep into the tissues.

In Āyurvedic medicine, four types of fats are indicated for internal consumption – ghee, oil, muscle fat, or bone marrow fat. Today, only ghee and oil are typically used because they are most appropriate for prevalent health conditions, readily available and easier to consume. Muscle fat and marrow fat are classically indicated for individuals who lead extremely active lives and are exceptionally strong with a high stress tolerance, which is rare today.

Ghee is considered to be an exceptional substance for strengthening the power of digestion (*agni*) while simultaneously encouraging *pitta doṣha* to operate within its normal range. Ghee is processed traditionally from fresh milk which is boiled, and then fermented into yogurt. From this, butter is churned, and heated to separate the solid whey from the clear, butter fat which is ghee. When used for medicinal compounding, ghee is stated to be "*saṁskāra anuvartana*" which means that it maintains its own specific properties while also assimilating properties of other medicinal substances during processing. This creates a powerful medicinal compound that effectively resets digestion, normalizes *pitta*, and can target specific conditions based on additional ingredients.

With ghee and oil, many options are available. These start with plain, unprocessed ghee and oil products that are available at many supermarkets and span to include complex formulations of processed and compounded herbal-infused products. Neither end of the spectrum is necessarily better or worse than the other. The choice to use regular ghee or oil, or herbal-infused ghee or oil completely depends on the individual, their state of health, the intention of the Complete Virechana, and whatever is safest and most effective for the situation. Your Āyurveda Āchārya will determine which option is best for you based on your assessments, goals, limitations and any potential complications.

Stage 2 requires a minimum of three days and maximum limit of seven days. There is no "normal" number of days as reaching the correct outcome varies based on each individual, their digestive power, capacity and current state of health or disease. There can be an anticipated number of days specific to an individual, and that prediction typically increases in accuracy on a subsequent Complete Virechana.

For your first experience, it is always best to mentally prepare yourself to be flexible during this part of the process because it is the most important stage of the entire procedure and responsible for overall outcome and positive improvements over the weeks and months that follow.

Each day, your Āyurveda Āchārya will determine whether to continue in Stage 2 or move on to the next stage based on how much fat was consumed, how the digestive system, body and mind responded, and how the rest of the day went. While it may be possible to estimate how many days will be required for Stage 2, always remember that it is likely to change.

There are a set of signs that specifically indicate whether to continue consuming fats or to stop and those can only be assessed by your Āyurveda Āchārya each day during this stage. Expect to discuss and review your experience each day after the fat completely digests and you complete the rest of the activities that should follow (detailed next). Your Āyurveda Āchārya will let you know when to expect to check-in each day. That time usually moves later and later each day during Stage 2 because of the length of time needed for complete digestion.

General procedure

The procedure followed during Stage 2 will remain mostly the same for the full stage, so it should be relatively easy to get into the routine of it. The first day may take a little longer as you get comfortable with doing each of the tasks carefully and accurately, but it will become noticeably easier on subsequent days. Typically, it takes about 10-15 minutes to prepare the fat and hot water to drink, and to be able to sit down comfortably and consume it.

Do not eat or drink anything else before consuming your dose of fat for the day during Stage 2. Do not even drink hot water before the fat. The fat must be the very first thing that enters into the digestive system for it to work properly.

The ideal wake up time during this stage is 30 to 60 minutes before sunrise, which should be no later than 7 am. The ideal time of year for Complete Virechana is typically at the end of the summer in temperate zones. In tropical and subtropical zones that experience a monsoon or hurricane season, Complete Virechana may be more appropriate towards the end of the rainy season when the sun and heat reemerge.

In locales or seasons where the sun rises later than 7 am, ask your Āyurveda Āchārya for specific instructions on times to wake up and prepare for consuming ghee.

If you wake up more than 120 minutes before sunrise, you should stay in bed and allow yourself to doze off if still feeling tired. Do not do any activities, or only do something that is boring and will help you feel sleepy.

If you wake up between 60 to 120 minutes before sunrise, do not try to fall asleep again. You can stay in bed if feeling tired, weak or exhausted, which is normal especially going further into the Complete Virechana. Rest, stay warm and listen to something calming. You can practice meditation or spiritual activities focusing on gratitude, optimism and visualization.

If you wake up between 30 to 60 minutes before sunrise, just get up. Go to the bathroom, relieve any urge to urinate, defecate or release gas, then wash the hands and rinse the face with warm water. Brush the teeth and rinse the mouth with warm water. After completing your morning hygiene routine, perform an early morning initial assessment.

Early morning initial assessment

Each morning upon waking and rising, you will be asked to perform a self-assessment to look for signs and symptoms of digestion of fat. In the first few days, these signs may change subtly. As you progress, certain signs should become strongly apparent.

Recognizing these signs and recording them is extremely important to the successful outcome of Complete Virechana whether performing the procedure at home or in a facility. You are ultimately responsible for communicating these details to your Āyurveda Āchārya and Svastha Āchārya. Be sure to record them daily, preferably first thing in the morning, when you are able to clearly assess them.

You should be observant of anything you notice that feels unusual and anything that has changed in the following areas:

1. Physical body – sensations of pain, temperature, stiffness, heaviness, lightness, or others
2. Mental, emotional disposition – thoughts, tendencies, behaviors, enthusiasm
3. Digestion – elimination, hunger levels, energy levels
4. Disease or dysfunction – signs or symptoms of existing disease, pre-disease or abnormality

You can use any tracking tools provided by your Āyurveda Āchārya or note details in your records in the Appendix. Be as descriptive as possible and monitor signs and symptoms daily.

Fat preparation

1. Begin fat preparation at least 30 minutes before sunrise on the first day.
2. On subsequent days as you become more comfortable with this, you may only need 15 to 20 minutes to prepare the fat and hot water.
3. Prepare freshly boiled water to drink along with the fat. Pour some hot water in a glass so that it has reached a drinkable temperature once the fat is heated and ready. This is done first so the water temperature is just right after the fat is consumed.

4. In a separate, medium pot, put 1-3 cups of plain tap water on high heat and bring to a boil. This water will not be used for drinking. The amount of water to boil depends on how you plan to heat the ghee. There should be enough water to let the measuring glass sit in the hot water without falling over.
5. While the water is heating, get a clean, dry measuring glass and metal spoon along with your specific fat for drinking. Shake or stir the fat to mix it consistently if you notice any separation.
6. Measure the amount of fat to be used for the day. See the details in the next section for your specific daily amount as directed by the Āyurveda Āchārya. If instructed, add a tiny pinch of pink crystal salt.
7. If using ghee, remember that in its un-melted state, it will not measure accurately. Most likely, you will need to put a portion of the amount in the glass measuring cup, heat it, and then add the remaining to get an accurate measurement. Also remember that the amount of ghee left on the spoon can add to the final quantity.
8. When the ghee melts, if there is too much in the glass, move it back to the original container by ladling it with the spoon. Do not try to pour it.
9. Whether you're using oil or ghee, the final measurement should be made where the meniscus meets the gradient mark on the measuring cup, as shown next.

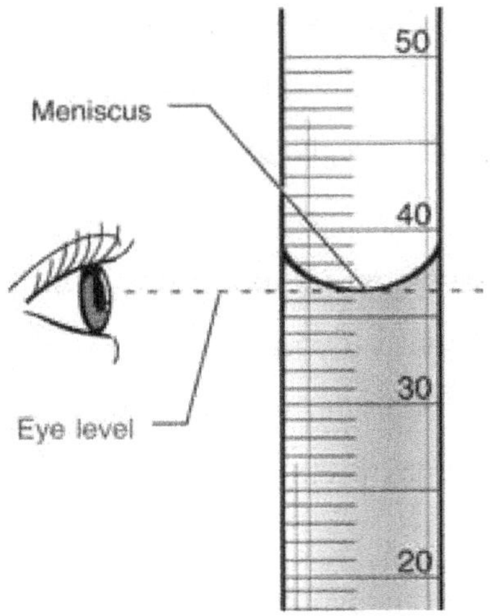

10. To heat the fat, always remove the boiled water from heat first. Either place the measuring cup directly into the pot of boiled water, or pour the hot water into a separate glass bowl and then place the measuring cup into the bowl. The bowl method is safer as it will be easier to control the water level, and to place and remove the measuring glass. Always place the measuring glass into the hot water slowly and carefully as sudden changes in temperature can cause brittle glass to crack.
11. Do not allow any moisture to contaminate the fat while it is heating.
12. Use the spoon to carefully stir the fat so it is mixed consistently. Make sure to steady the measuring glass as you do this so that it does not tip over and spill.
13. Test the temperature of the fat very carefully by checking the heat of the spoon and by watching for changes in the fat's viscosity as it heats. As it becomes thinner, you can understand that it is becoming warmer. The ideal temperature for drinking fats is just above body temperature, but never so hot that it could burn the lips, mouth or throat. It is best to heat the fat to a slightly

higher point than you will use for drinking because it is easier to find the correct, comfortable temperature as it cools.

14. If the hot water is not sufficient to heat the fat completely, you may need to empty it and refill it with freshly boiled hot water.
15. Once the fat is ready, remove it from the hot water carefully using an oven mitt, towel or other utensil that can handle hot glass.
16. Dry the outside of the measuring glass and wrap it in a towel to make it easy to hold while you drink.

Alternatively, the fat can be heated in the glass measuring cup by placing it directly on a heating element that is set to its lowest temperature. This method is more risky as the glass may crack or overheat more easily. If you want to use this heating option, be sure to discuss the method with your Āyurveda Āchārya or Svastha Āchārya so you can perform it safely.

Consuming the prepared fat

1. Take the measuring glass with the heated fat and the cup of hot water to drink and set them down where you plan to consume them.
2. Sit in a chair which is comfortable, and neither too large or too small. Ideally, you should be able to sit back with good support, and still be able to rest your feet flat on the ground without feeling undue pressure on the thighs or backs of the knees. For some people, a small stool with a sitting cushion placed next to a wall may be the best option. Make sure that the seat has enough padding or cushion so that the sit bones are not uncomfortable on a hard or cold surface. If needed, cover yourself with a blanket to stay warm.
3. Do not stand, lay down or sit in a slouched, relaxed position for consuming the fat. The spine needs to be straight and well-supported to allow the digestive tract to function properly.

4. If possible, position your seat to face east where you can look out a window. It is ideal to observe the rising sun while consuming the fat. This is the optimal timing in classical practice.
5. When you are comfortably positioned and ready, take the heated fat in the measuring cup and first press the towel against the lip of the glass where you plan to drink from. This removes some excess heat and helps prevent burning the lips on contact with the glass. Always check the glass temperature carefully first with a fingertip or back side of a finger and then briefly test it near the lips to make sure that it is not too hot.
6. Once the glass temperature is checked correctly, next check the temperature of the fat to make sure it is comfortably hot. Tilt the fat towards the lips and try to gauge the temperature first without actually touching the fat to the lips. If it is extremely hot you will be able to feel it at this point. If it is not too hot, try touching the fat to the lips to determine if it is the right temperature for drinking.
7. If the fat is not hot enough, it must be reheated before continuing.
8. Once you know that it is the right temperature, start drinking. The goal is to finish the full quantity while it is hot and avoid vomiting. Some people like to sip the fat slowly, while others prefer to down the entire thing at once, even for large doses. Find out what works for you and finish drinking it as quickly as you can.
9. If the temperature becomes too cold to drink at any point, the fat will need to be reheated. This should be avoided as it creates an interruption and delays the drinking time. For larger doses, it may be unavoidable, so be prepared to reheat if you expect that you'll consume it slowly.
10. If drinking the fat suddenly makes you feel nauseous, take a few deep breaths and try taking a sip or two of very hot water to wash it down. Resume drinking the fat as soon as possible to avoid delays. To reduce the sensation of nausea, smell the rind of a lemon after scratching the surface to open it. The strong fragrance will help alleviate nausea.
11. After consuming the entire quantity of fat, take a few sips of hot water to help wash it down.

12. If you feel a continued sense of nausea, use the hot water to rinse your mouth and gargle several times. Take deep breaths and either sit very still or walk very slowly in a straight line back and forth (not in a circle). Make every attempt to control the nausea but if it becomes uncontrollable, do vomit. If this happens you should contact the Āyurveda Āchārya immediately for instructions.
13. In most cases, especially on the initial days with a lower dose, the fat goes down and stays down easily. In this case, you can either sit for a few minutes in the same position with a straight back and sip on hot water or you can walk slowly to encourage digestive movement.
14. After about 15-20 minutes you may notice the urge to urinate. Whenever this urge manifests you should immediately go to the bathroom and release it.

After consuming fat (digestion phase)

1. Once the fat has been completely consumed and it is clear that it will be kept down without issue, you are in the digestion phase.
2. While the fat is digesting, you will notice certain signs from the digestive system that it is being processed. These signs can include burps, changes in energy and mental state, various noises from the gut, release of waste materials, and several more common symptoms that are detailed next. You will need to be aware of these signs throughout the entire digestion phase. Observe them, track them and record them in your journal or records. If using an electronic journal with your Āyurveda Āchārya, you may type the information in directly at this time as long as it does not induce a sense of nausea. If looking at a screen feels uncomfortable while the ghee is digesting, write your observations down on paper and enter them later.
3. It is natural to feel drowsy, tired and exhausted while the fat is digesting because it is extremely heavy. But it is imperative that you do not fall asleep at any point during the day. You should make every attempt to avoid feeling sleepy by getting up frequently and slowly walking around

the house to keep the body slightly active and encourage normal circulation. Plan to get up and walk around at least once every 30 minutes.

4. You must also continue to sip on hot water to encourage complete digestion of the fat. Plan to consume about 1 cup of water each hour spaced out as needed. Sip it gradually, or drink about a quarter cup every 15 minutes or a half a cup every half hour. Make sure that the water is always piping hot. You can keep freshly boiled hot water ready in a flask and pour just the amount that you want to drink at that time.
5. Never use leftover boiled water from the previous day. Each day you should boil fresh, hot drinking water every few hours so it does not become stale.
6. At any point, if you feel the urge to pass urine, bowels or gas, do so immediately. Do not delay or hold it for even a few minutes. This also applies to any other urges, natural reflexes, or natural bodily responses, including burping, coughing, crying, etc.
7. Activities during the digestion phase can vary widely, and have been discussed to some extent in the earlier sections on Preparation and Planning. You must determine what feels right to engage yourself in at the time, keeping in mind that this can vary from day to day especially as the quantity of fat increases.
8. The simplest activity is to sit in a chair covered with blankets and stare out a window at a natural scene. This allows you the best chance to observe what the body and mind are doing in this resting state. It is the best thing to do immediately after consuming fats to allow the body to direct all of its energy towards digestion. Simple, non-engaging activities like this should be continued until the fat has completely digested.
9. If you feel cold or have a difficult time maintaining a warm body temperature consistently, sit under blankets with a hot water bottle or heating pack for 30-60 minutes at a time. Once you feel warm and possibly sweaty, do not rush to remove layers. Instead, just remove the heating

pack and continue to stay bundled up sufficiently to maintain a proper temperature. Good thermogenesis (generation of bodily heat) encourages correct processing of the consumed fat.

10. Light walking or gentle ambulation is encouraged for short periods inside the home, facility or premises, without being exposed to direct sunlight, breeze or any uncomfortable elements.
11. On the days where fat quantity is higher, digestion time will definitely take longer. On these days you may need to engage yourself in some very light, stress-free activities to pass the time. These activities can be great for short periods (20-30 minutes at a time, not more) as long as they keep the mind in a peaceful, positive state and do not inflict any type of stress. Light reading, looking at pictures, watching nature shows on television, painting, drawing, etc. can all be beneficial for short periods, interspersed with disconnecting from them and getting up for gentle walking.
12. Interactions with other people should be avoided during fat digestion. Too much talking, over stimulation, excessive concentration or fluctuations in emotions can cause unnecessary stress and disruption that detracts from digestion.
13. You might be asked to drink ginger tea, or ginger-coriander tea to aid digestion on certain days. Typically, this is made by adding one-quarter teaspoon of the powder to a full cup of freshly boiled hot water, mixing, and allowing to steep. Let the powder sink to the bottom of the cup and sip on it while hot. This tea should be finished while hot, and should not be reheated.

Assessing fat digestion

There are specific criteria for determining whether the fat has digested completely or not. These can be checked roughly every half to one hour, knowing that it takes an absolute minimum of 3 hours for any amount of fat to get digested.

Use this guide each day to determine how long the fat takes to digest completely. Ideally, all the assessment criteria should be present to some degree to ensure full digestion. Your Āyurveda Āchārya will perform this assessment with you each day and answer any questions you have.

Record the length of time for digestion each day in your daily record or tracker.

Assessment criteria	**Explanation**
Clear burps	True burps that present naturally (not by swallowing air intentionally) should be completely clear and free of any taste, especially taste of the fat. This should happen continuously, and not be interspersed with burps that do have any remnant flavor.
Enthusiasm	Enthusiasm in this context will be noticed as a slightly higher level of energy and interest in being active, compared to the levels in the first few hours after consuming the fat. Considering the context, expect your enthusiasm to be less than what it might be on a normal day. It may even seem more like a sense of contentment or satisfaction, or eagerness and happiness about yourself and your current situation.
Proper downward movement of wastes	All wastes which are normally expelled downwards (urine, feces and gas) should be moving easily and unimpeded in their normal pathways. There should be no feeling of obstruction, blockage, sluggishness or absence of movement in the GIT, especially in the area at and below the navel.
Lightness	This can be easily recognized as the opposite of the heavy feeling that would have been very obvious immediately after consuming the fat. You should feel light both physically and mentally, free of stress and tension, mobile and active.
Hunger	A clear, obvious and very recognizable feeling of hunger should be present. If hunger sensations like rumbling in the stomach, increased salivation, and desire to eat arise but only when thinking of favorite foods or seeing food,

	wait at least 15 minutes before assuming that it is a true manifestation of hunger. Continue to sip on hot water and monitor any burps. Eating too soon (before the fat has fully digested) is the easiest and quickest way to create complications in the entire process.
Thirst	It may be difficult to gauge genuine thirst because you will be frequently sipping on hot water. But after correct digestion of the fat, hunger and thirst will generally appear together. Watch for subtle signs of an increased feeling of dryness in the throat, nose or eyes, and a reduction in saliva. Towards the end of fat digestion, start to increase the quantity of hot water and reduce the frequency. This will help confirm that the fat has digested.

After fat digestion is complete

Once it is clear that the fat from the morning has completely digested, follow these steps.

1. Start preparing congee for one to two servings. Either wash and let the rice soak while taking a shower, or put it on to gently simmer. Do not leave it cooking unattended if it may boil over. You can also bring it to a boil, shut it off, and turn it on again once you're finished showering. This will allow it to cook faster.
2. Empty the bladder and bowels, if any urge is present.
3. Take a warm to hot shower using mild shampoo and soap with slightly less than you normally would use. If absolutely necessary, a very small amount of conditioner is allowable but only on the tips of the hair and not on the scalp. Be sure to rinse all products off of the body completely. The water temperature should be comfortably hot, at or around body temperature, and never too hot or too cold. Stay in the shower only long enough to finish washing, and not so long that the fingertips begin to prune. Only showers are allowed at this point in the process, no baths.

4. Do not apply any other products, lotions, creams, beauty care items, oils or anything at all to the skin after showering. Just dry off quickly after getting out of the shower and get dressed.
5. Put on clean clothes that are preferably natural fiber material, with long sleeves and long pants. Always wear whatever clothing is appropriate or necessary to maintain a consistently warm body temperature that is borderline sweating. For some, this might require wearing multiple layers, hats, socks and slippers. Use as much as you need to feel warm and cozy. During this stage, you must stay fully covered unless you are in a tropical, hot and humid environment.
6. Rest immediately after getting dressed. Cover yourself with blankets if needed and have some hot water to drink nearby. If necessary, turn the congee on to cook while you rest.
7. Drink a half to full cup of hot water (or whatever quantity feels filling) and wait up to 30 minutes to observe how it is digesting. If you notice any burps that taste like the fat, it has not completely digested yet.
8. Check-in with your digestion progress again and confirm that all signs indicate that the fat has fully digested. If not, rest a little longer or walk around slowly and continue to sip on hot water.
9. When the fat has completely digested, eat your first bowl of congee. This must be freshly-made, soupy, not too thick and seasoned only with a low amount of pink crystal salt. Use the recipe in Recovery meal #3 or follow your specific instructions.
10. To eat your bowl of congee, make sure you're sitting in a comfortable position where the feet can rest firmly on the floor. Avoid any distractions, like television, computer or smartphone, and concentrate only on eating. Also avoid conversation unless it is limited and allows you to remain attentive to eating. Focus on each bite, eating neither too quickly nor too slowly. Take sips of hot water in between bites if you feel thirsty.
11. Once you notice that you feel full, usually accompanied by a burp or two, stop eating, even if you have not finished the full bowl. Never overeat during this process at it can lead to indigestion and complications.

12. If you’ve prepared extra congee, you can save one more serving for later the same day. However, it must be stored on the counter and not in the fridge. It can stay good for about 4 to 6 hours in temperate climates. If an extra serving ever seems questionable with an odd smell, color, taste or texture, do not eat it and instead prepare a fresh batch.

Stage 3, Mobilization

Preparatory stage (*pūrva karma*) to loosen the *doșhas*, with external oil massage and steam bath (*bāhya snehana* and *svedana*)

Purpose and duration

Once your Āyurveda Āchārya determines that Stage 2 is complete, you will move on to Stage 3. This is often considered to be the best part of Complete Virechana. It features the external body treatments of oil massage (*abhyaṅga*) followed by a steam bath (*svedana*) and hot shower. The combination is soothing, relaxing, comforting and relieving, especially after consuming fat.

This stage includes the treatments which are typically portrayed as spa activities (under the guise of Pañcha Karma) showing relaxed, happy, and usually beautiful women laying on a massage table being pampered with oil.

In residential facilities under the direct supervision of an Āyurveda Āchārya, these treatments are performed by same-sex therapists only. This supports full relaxation during the procedure to experience maximum benefits.

Stage 3 has its own routine and schedule which is followed for 3 days in a row immediately after the completion of Stage 2. The goal during Stage 3 is to lubricate the body externally using the combination of oil through massage followed by steam heat in an enclosed chamber to induce sweating. Both of these treatments must be done together in this specified order to achieve the desired results.

The external lubrication of the body and softening of the tissues with steam heat allows waste materials (*doșhas*) which are stuck in the tissues to exude out into circulation. During Stage 2, the consumption of fat penetrates the body's tissue layers internally allowing the fat to bind to waste materials (*doșhas*) which are either hidden or lodged in various tissues.

In Stage 3, the external application of oil with massage helps to gently loosen the lodged waste materials (*doṣhas*) from their hiding spots. Then, heating the body encourages minute but sufficient expansion between the tissues. Coupled with increased circulation and perfusion, the result is the loosening and detachment of waste material from normal, healthy bodily tissues.

Stage 3 also allows several additional and significant events to take place before the actual elimination happens on Virechana day in Stage 4. Fat consumption naturally causes an increase in the quantity and qualities of heavy waste materials like mucus and phlegm (related to *kapha doṣha*) in the body which can obstruct elimination. The dislodged heavy waste materials (*kapha doṣha*) tend to exit through the upper route rather than the lower route, which must be avoided during Virechana.

Therefore, in Āyurvedic medicine it is a requirement to wait three full days and nights in between the final digestion of the fat on the last day of Stage 2 and the actual elimination day of Stage 4. These three days are reserved for external treatments to help reduce the load of *kapha doṣha* waste materials from the tissues. Allowing *kapha doṣha* to normalize is key to a successful Virechana with downward elimination rather than upward.

General procedure

During Stage 3, you should continue to wake up at the same time each day as you had been waking up during Stage 2 in order to keep the body's circadian rhythm, hormones and endocrine system firmly established in a healthy routine. Immediately after waking, head to the bathroom and empty the bladder and bowels if any urge is present. Wash the hands with warm water and rinse the face with tepid water. Rinse the mouth, expel any phlegm from the throat and brush the teeth.

Boil fresh water and pour a small cup to sip on. For these mornings, you can do very basic and simple movement activities to lengthen and stretch the body soon after getting up. Slow, controlled and non-stressful routines often seen in Tai Chi are ideal. Certain Yoga Āsanas are allowed as long as they do not increase the heart rate or breathing rate excessively. Any gentle movement done during this time should be so easy that it doesn't break a sweat. Generally, you will not take a shower first thing in the morning since you will have one after the treatments.

Depending on your overall level of strength, state of digestion and metabolism (*agni*), the external body treatments of oil massage (*abhyaṅga*) and steam bath (*svedana*) might be performed before or a few hours after your first meal. In rare cases, your treatments may be performed in the afternoon after lunch. However, treatments are never performed at night. The oil massage (*abhyaṅga*) will include a head massage and a copious amount of oil over the entire body.

After the oil massage and steam bath, you'll take a shower with warm water that is not too hot. Then you'll dry off, get dressed in warm clothing with long sleeves and rest for up to an hour. This will be followed by a meal of congee when you're feeling hungry. You should sip on freshly boiled hot water while resting.

Over the course of the entire day, expect to eat two or three meals of congee. Or, you may be instructed to eat a light soup which is easy-to-digest and not aggravating to any of the *doṣhas*. If your oil massage and steam treatments happen after eating, you'll need to wait at least an hour from the end of the meal before you start the treatment.

Your Āyurveda Āchārya will inform you about your schedule each day in advance. Be sure to note down your expected times for meals and treatments in your records in the Appendix.

If you are performing Complete Virechana on yourself at home, your Āyurveda Āchārya will provide clear instructions on meal and treatment timing. Remember that you must plan your days well so that your meals are ready when you are hungry. You must also be able to perform the external body treatments of oil massage (*abhyaṅga*) and steam bath (*svedana*) on yourself each day.

This will be difficult even if you are accustomed to doing these treatments because you will be weak and easily exhausted from moving and applying continuous pressure over your body. Do not strain yourself during the treatments and instead just stay relaxed. It is more important that the oil remain on your body for the full 45 minutes, and less important that you massage vigorously. Instead, just rub your body gently and slowly without overexerting yourself. After 45 minutes, get into the steam tent and sweat comfortably. Then take a warm to hot shower that keeps you warm to hot while you apply shampoo and soap to wash. Ideally, you should feel like you're sweating in the shower a little bit. After showering, dry off quickly, bundle up in warm clothes, sit comfortably under blankets, drink more hot water, and encourage your body to sweat while you rest.

Self-treatments

During Stage 3 and Stage 4, use these instructions to complete all self-treatments in order, at the time of day instructed by your Āyurveda Āchārya. If you are doing Complete Virechana in a facility, your Āyurveda Āchārya may change this timing and should inform you of your schedule on the prior day.

If you are doing Complete Virechana at home, expect to do your self-treatments at the same time each day during Stage 3 and possibly earlier during Stage 4. Ideally, these should all be done first thing in the morning, before eating anything.

The self-treatments include

1. Head massage (*śhiro abhyaṅga*)
2. Full-body oil massage (*abhyaṅga*)
3. Steam treatment to induce sweating (*svedana*)
4. Full shower, with shampoo and soap
5. Rest period

Head massage (*śhiro abhyaṅga*)

Applying oil to the scalp and combing it through the hair provides lubrication and nourishment to the micro channels of skin and underlying structures. It helps to allow waste products in the hair roots and follicles to pass out of the body more easily and effectively. Over time, regular oil application to the scalp and hair strengthens the hair shafts, promotes shine, softness and durability.

Timing

Ideal timing: Early morning, before breakfast

Duration: 5-10 minutes for application, 30-60 minutes for absorption

Applying oil to the scalp and massaging the head is best done early in the morning before eating anything. It should be followed by full-body *abhyaṅga*, and then showered out with shampoo.

Restrictions

Always avoid the following activities as they can produce side effects during or after the treatments.

- Do not apply oil to the scalp after consuming food. Wait until the food is completely digested, or at least four hours if unsure. If you do not feel hungry, contact your Āyurveda Āchārya and let them know.
- Do not apply oil to the scalp and leave it overnight. Oil must be washed out within two hours of initial application.
- Do not apply oil to the scalp and expose your body to any extreme temperatures, especially cold or breeze.
- Do not apply oil to the scalp and then eat anything before washing it out. If you feel very thirsty during the treatments, you can sip on hot water.

Procedure

From the time of starting the head massage, be prepared to spend about two hours on all treatments followed by a rest period.

1. Warm and melt the oil (if needed). Do not heat it excessively.
2. Shake the oil bottle to mix it well.
3. Part the hair to expose the scalp.

4. Apply the oil directly to the scalp. Massage it in with the fingertips directly to the scalp. The oil is most beneficial directly on the scalp, and less effective on the hair.
5. Repeat by parting other areas of the scalp and applying oil until the entire scalp has been lubricated.
6. Massage gently for a few minutes. For medium to longer hair, comb the oil through with a wide-toothed comb. Do not apply too much pressure to the scalp or scratch the scalp with the comb.
7. If desired, you can also massage the temples, around the ears and base of the skull along with the scalp.
8. Gently tie the hair back if desired, and let the oil sit for up to two hours.
9. Keep the body warm while the oil is on the scalp to prevent discomfort.
10. Shower and shampoo out completely.
11. Women should generally use warm (not too hot) water. Allow warm water to penetrate the hair completely for a few minutes before applying shampoo.
12. Men should generally use warm to tepid water that is definitely not hot. The water should not be too cold either as it will deactivate the sweating response which is required during this stage.
13. Do not apply conditioner.

Full-body oil massage (*abhyaṅga*)

Applying oil to the body along with massage provides lubrication and nourishment to the micro channels of the skin and underlying structures. It helps to allow waste products in the hair roots and follicles to pass out of the body more easily and effectively.

Over time, regular oil application to the body lubricates the skin and underlying structures, strengthens the channels of sweat to facilitate waste elimination and promotes cleaner, healthier functioning of underlying structures including the vascular and muscular systems.

Full-body oil application during this stage along with massage encourages waste materials in the tissues to dislodge into circulation for elimination in Stage 4.

Timing

Ideal timing: Early morning, before breakfast, immediately following head massage (*śhiro abhyaṅga*)

Duration: 5 minutes for application, 45 minutes for massage and absorption

Applying oil to the body and massaging it is best done early in the morning before eating anything. It should be done immediately following oil application to the scalp. After allowing the oil to absorb for 45 minutes, it must be followed by steam heat and then a warm to hot shower.

Restrictions

Always avoid the following activities as they can produce side effects during or after the treatments.

- Do not apply oil to the body after consuming food. Wait until the food is completely digested, or at least four hours if unsure. If you do not feel hungry, contact your Āyurveda Āchārya and let them know.
- Do not apply oil to the body and leave it on overnight. Oil must be washed off of the body within one hour of initial application.
- Do not apply oil to the body and expose your body to any extreme temperatures, especially cold or breeze.
- Do not apply oil to the body and then eat or drink anything before washing it off.

Procedure

From the time of starting the full-body oil application, be prepared to spend about one additional hour on remaining treatments followed by a rest period.

1. Warm and melt the oil, then shake the oil bottle to mix it well.
2. Be in a small room that is easy to keep warm (preferably the bathroom).
3. Stand on a towel to keep the feet warm and catch any oil when it drips.

4. Apply warm oil over the entire body. Gently apply oil to the face and neck, and rub oil into the nostrils and ears. If oil drips into the eyes and is uncomfortable, wipe it off gently with a soft towel.
5. Massage with circular movements over the middle of the body and joints with gentle pressure.
6. Massage with long strokes over the limbs with medium pressure and squeeze from the hands and feet towards the core.
7. Be sure to keep the oil on the entire body for 45 minutes. If it is too exhausting to massage yourself for the entire duration, rest instead. Ideally keep the body covered and warm with a bath robe or other garments. These will become very oily each day.

Steam treatment to induce sweating (*svedana*)

A steam heat treatment or application is generally done after head massage and full-body *abhyaṅga*. The damp heat allows the pores of the skin to open and flush, while simultaneously allowing the oil to penetrate the tissues more deeply. The benefits of these treatments only occur in this order, meaning that steam heat should always follow oil, and never be done in reverse. Oil should never be applied after steam or shower.

The goal of the steam heat treatment is to produce the right amount of sweat. This is indicated by the following signs:

1. Appearance (or feeling) of sweat, especially from areas that are not directly exposed to heat like the upper lip and forehead
2. Reduction of stiffness, heaviness and coldness

When performing this treatment, aim to expose yourself to the right amount of heat for just long enough to sweat and feel light, perky and awake. Always stop any heat treatment if it feels uncomfortable. Excess heat exposure can produce acute complications, fainting and in some cases a serious medical emergency.

Timing

Ideal timing: Early morning, before breakfast, immediately following full-body oil massage (*abhyaṅga*)

Duration: 30 minutes or less

Equipment

A steam heat treatment may be done in a steam tent, hot bath, or in the shower. Review the common options described below, and discuss your options with your Āyurveda Āchārya and Svastha Āchārya to determine what's best for you.

The head should not be exposed to heat during the treatment, unless recommended by your Āyurveda Āchārya. This prevents excessive build up of pressure in the skull which can adversely affect the eyes and sense organs.

You may be advised to use certain medicinal herbs as part of the steam heat treatment. These may include powders like *daśha-mūla, balā-mūla* or *eraṇḍa-mūla*.

Portable steam tent (search for "steam tent" on Amazon) – This is the ideal way to do a steam heat treatment because it allows the body to be bathed in warm steam. This is gentle yet highly effective with low risk of excess heat exposure. Products available online through Amazon and other vendors change quickly. Choose an option where the head can remain outside of the heat, unless recommended by your Āyurveda Āchārya. Expect the tent to get oily and sticky quickly, and require regular maintenance to keep it clean and well-functioning.

Hot bath – This is the most challenging way to do a heat treatment for several reasons. When covered in oil, it is very difficult to get in and out of a bathtub easily. There is a high risk for slipping and falling, and anyone who is prone to that should avoid this method. It can also be difficult to get the correct level of heat in the water. Start with a lower heat and then add more hot water once the body is adjusted. Do not submerge the body in excessively hot water as this can quickly aggravate many conditions and produce side effects or fainting.

Shower – This is the easiest way to do a heat treatment, however it usually provides the lowest level of heat. For some, it may be completely inadequate for producing sweating, or take a very long time. If this is your only method for a steam heat treatment, try to heat the bathroom up as much as possible first and enclose the shower space to retain steam and heat. Remain in the shower under moderately warm to hot water for as long as possible. Do not use excessively hot water that produces goosebumps as this is a sign of other underlying metabolic conditions that will be aggravated by excessive heat.

Restrictions

Always avoid the following activities as they can produce side effects during or after the treatments.

- Do not perform a steam heat treatment after consuming food. Wait until the food is completely digested, or at least four hours if unsure. If you do not feel hungry, contact your Āyurveda Āchārya and let them know.
- Do not perform a steam heat treatment without applying oil to the body first, unless specifically instructed by your Āyurveda Āchārya.
- For one hour after a steam heat treatment, do not expose your body to any extreme temperatures, especially cold or any breeze.
- Do not overexpose yourself to heat during this treatment at any time or for any duration. This can cause fainting or other complications.
- After a steam heat treatment, avoid eating for at least 60 minutes. If thirsty and not overheated, drink warm or hot water. If thirsty and overheated, immediately drink cool, room temperature water and contact your Āyurveda Āchārya for further instructions.

Procedure

Perform a steam heat treatment after a head massage and full-body *abhyaṅga*. Then, follow it with a shower and rest period.

1. First, set up the steam tent or other equipment that will be used for the steam heat treatment. Make sure everything is functioning properly at least one day in advance to ensure that you are comfortable operating the equipment.
2. If using medicinal herbs with the steam generator, include the powder(s) in the steam heating unit. If necessary, enclose them in a muslin cloth bag so they do not clog the tubing while the generator is switched on.
3. Prepare the head and body by properly applying oil for the full duration of time.
4. Turn the steam heat equipment on so that it is producing heat. Let it warm and preferably fill the tent with steam prior to getting inside.
5. Sit, lie or stand in the equipment. Keep the head outside of the equipment or cover the head with a damp towel to avoid or reduce direct exposure to heat.
6. Relax as much as possible in the heat.
7. Observe the signs and symptoms during the course of the treatment. Constantly monitor the following as sensations that you feel internally and by touching different parts of your body.
    a. Relief from cold, increase in warmth and heat
    b. Reduction of bodily and joint stiffness, increase in ease of mobility
    c. Appearance of sweat
8. Note the progression of signs and symptoms over the period of heat application so you can record them in your journal or tracker after the treatments.
9. If the head is outside of the heat, notice when sweat appears over the upper lip, forehead or face. If you feel comfortably hot and sweaty when this appears, stop the heat within a few minutes or as soon as you feel you've had enough.

10. Also notice changes in energy levels, feelings of discomfort or irritability, and stop the heat if any of these appear.
11. Otherwise, stop the heat around the 25 minute mark.
12. Once the heat has stopped, rest for one to two minutes before slowly get out of the equipment.
13. Proceed directly to take a hot shower.

Full shower, with shampoo and soap

After head massage (*śhiro-abhyaṅga*), full-body oil application (*abhyaṅga*) and steam heat treatment (*svedana*), the body must be cleaned properly so that the excess oil and adhered waste products are removed. Use a moderate to strong shampoo and lather well to remove the oil from the scalp and hair. Do not apply conditioner.

For the body, use a mild soap, herbal powder, or salt scrub to remove the excess oil and adhered wastes. Depending on the skin's tendency to be oily or dry, use the appropriate amount of soap or cleanser to remove all of the oil (using more soap) or leave enough to keep the skin moisturized (using less soap). If desired, you can use a wash cloth, bath sponge or gentle loofa along with the soap. Alternatively, use just your hands and gently rub and squeeze the tissues to work the oil and soap into the skin for deeper cleansing.

Herbal powder can be made from dry-roasted moong dal (including the husk), which is powdered. However, this can easily clog smaller drains and create expensive plumbing issues.

If you are using a shower for the steam heat treatment (*svedana*) following oil application, the shower must produce enough heat to warm the body to the point of sweating. This will generally require a much longer shower of 20 to 30 minutes or more, in some cases. Do not use excessively hot water to try to induce sweating as this will cause side effects and complications.

Showers during Complete Virechana should always use water that is warm to hot. Water must be at least as hot as body temperature, and preferably slightly warmer. It should never be cooler than body temperature, nor should it be very hot.

Water applied to the head should be warm, around body temperature, especially for women. For men, it should be slightly cooler than body temperature, but neither too cold nor too hot.

After showering, get out and dry off quickly in the warm bathroom. Get dressed immediately with as many layers as needed to retain the heat and promote continued warmth and a gentle sweat for at least 30 minutes. Sit comfortably under blankets and sip on hot water. Rest for about 30 minutes or until feeling hungry, then have the appropriate meal.

Special preparation for Virechana day

On the third night of Stage 3, you may be asked to have one special preparation drink about an hour before you go to bed. Be sure to check with your Āyurveda Āchārya on the third day to find out if this is recommended.

If your Āyurveda Āchārya advises it, use the following instructions.

1. Bring one cup of water to a full boil.
2. Pour the water into a cup and let it cool so that you can drink it, but it is still warm.
3. Squeeze about ¼ to ½ of a Meyer's lemon into the water. If you cannot get a Meyer's lemon, use a fully ripened, regular lime.
4. Add a tiny pinch of salt to the water.
5. Mix everything well.
6. Drink the entire cup while hot or warm.

This preparation drink helps to excite *pitta* throughout the body so that the formulations in Stage 4 can be more effective. It will encourage the excited *pitta* to move into the gastrointestinal tract so that it can be eliminated the following day.

Stage 4, Elimination

Operative stage to eliminate the *doṣhas* (*pradhāna karma*), with therapeutic purgation (*virechana*)

Purpose and duration

After three full days of Stage 3, it is time to move to Stage 4: Elimination. This is a standard time period in Complete Virechana and should not be shortened or extended.

Stage 4: Elimination, normally consists of just one day. It includes an early morning set of all treatments, followed by a short rest. Then the formulations are administered and bowel movements generally begin in one to two hours. Bowel movements typically last most of the day. Expect to take a shower towards the end of the day and eat one small meal of congee water with very mild flavoring.

In some rare cases, a second day is required during Stage 4: Elimination. This can be due to a number of factors like unfavorable conditions in the external environment, insufficient dosing of the formulation(s), incompatibility of the formulation(s) for the individual, or other unforeseen circumstances.

If you require a second day in Stage 4, your Āyurveda Āchārya will discuss this with you on the first day and explain the reasons why. If performing Complete Virechana at home, you will work with your Āyurveda Āchārya to decide how to proceed based on your specific circumstances.

Preparing for purgation

During Stage 4, wake up around the same time that you had been waking in the previous stages. This should be about an hour before sunrise. Get up, go to the bathroom and do your morning hygiene and put fresh water on to boil. Drink one to two cups of freshly boiled hot water and gently move or stretch the body, if you feel up for it.

Next, perform your self-treatments in the same way as you did on the previous days in Stage 3. These include head massage (*śhiro abhyaṅga*), full-body oil massage (*abhyaṅga*), steam treatment to induce sweating (*svedana*) and a full shower with shampoo and soap followed by a rest period. Continue to sip on freshly boiled hot water during the rest period and stay comfortable, warm and almost sweating.

Plan your treatments so that you finish everything, including the rest period, between 9 am to 9:15 am. The latest time to finish is 9:30 am.

Formulations and fluids

Between 9 am and 9:30 am, you will consume the formulations that will induce therapeutic purgation as bouts of bowel movements. Your Āyurveda Āchārya will provide instructions on which formulations to take, how much to use, how to prepare them and how to consume them. Always use a digital scale to measure the formulations unless otherwise specified.

The formulations are designed to expel dislodged waste materials from the body by bringing them into the digestive tract via circulation. Remember that during Stage 3: Lubrication, the waste products were detached from their locations throughout the body and allowed to enter circulation. The formulations in Stage 4 work directly on those mobilized waste products and bring them into the digestive tract so that they can be eliminated through the correct channel. In this case, it is via downward elimination through the rectum as bowel movements.

To produce this effectively and for the quantum of waste products dislodged in the previous stages, the formulations often produce a sense of discomfort. This is normal as long as it is within a tolerable range that includes symptoms like moderate nausea but not vomiting, slight headaches, tiredness and weakness, gurgling and movement in the intestines, and an overall feeling of general sickness.

Keep a fresh lemon ready in case you begin to feel uncomfortable, queasy or nauseous while consuming the formulations. Scratch the rind and sniff the fresh scent of the lemon. This will help alleviate some of the nausea. You can continue to do this as needed for two hours after consuming the formulations.

All signs and symptoms should be reported to your Āyurveda Āchārya. Keep a record of what you feel and experience, when and its intensity. Discuss these when you check in with your Āyurveda Āchārya.

If any signs and symptoms become excessively uncomfortable, or if you experience vomiting, intense cramping or pain, bowel movements with blood or other unknown components, notify your Āyurveda Āchārya immediately. In rare cases, allergic reactions to formulations can occur. These may require emergency medical attention.

If at any time you experience a medical emergency during Stage 4, call for help immediately, or go directly to an emergency medical center. Have your emergency plan ready along with any medical documents and be prepared to use them if needed.

Expect bowel movements to begin about 30 to 120 minutes after consuming the formulations. Use the checklist below to encourage easy flow of bowel movements and minimize complications. If nothing has happened within two hours following the formulations, contact your Āyurveda Āchārya.

Continue to drink freshly boiled hot water after the formulations and throughout the entire day so that you consume two to four liters total. Boil water in one half liter or liter increments, and store it in a flask or container. Record how many containers you consume and the time completed. Be sure to note this information in your journal or tracker.

After consuming the formulations, be sure to monitor and manage the following.

1. **Stay warm**. Check your skin on your face, cheeks, nose and ears for temperature. Check your extremities, including fingers and toes. If any of these feel cool to touch, and your core temperature is not very warm and about to sweat, the bowel movements may not begin. The body must reach a sufficiently high operating temperature for bowel movements to begin flowing. Add more layers, increase the ambient temperature or use a water bottle or heating pad to increase your core temperature.
2. **Stay hydrated**. You should consume around one full liter of freshly boiled hot water within two hours after the formulations. This can include the total hot water that you had for the entire day, including before and after the treatments. Avoid over-hydrating and do not force water

excessively especially if feeling nauseous. Sip on it or drink it in larger quantities as you feel able to without worsening any symptoms.

3. **Stay mobile**. Move around gently whenever possible. Walk slowly around the house or premises every 10 to 15 minutes. Sit in a comfortable but firm chair that allows your pelvis and spine to remain in good alignment. Avoid slouching or bad posture as this can impede circulatory flow and intestinal movement.
4. **Stay attentive**. Notice any urges to pass urine, gas or the bowels. Make sure to attend to these as soon possible even if it doesn't feel that strong. Allowing urine and gas to move down and out easily promotes general downward flow and encourages the body to begin eliminating bowel movements.

If bowel movements have not started within two hours after consuming the formulations, contact your Āyurveda Āchārya and discuss next steps.

Purgation and bowel movements

Once the bowel movements begin, they will usually continue on their own until the formulations have exhausted themselves. However, you must continue to be aware of the points noted above and stay warm, stay hydrated, stay mobile and stay attentive to keep things moving smoothly and easily throughout the day.

Bouts typically continue for 6 to 12 hours and will mostly consist of water or fluid. Initially, there may be some stool material in the first one or two bouts of elimination, but that will quickly change over to more fluid with less contents.

It is ideal to use a bidet to wash the area after each bowel movement. Then it can be dried by lightly tapping with toilet paper. It is not recommended to wipe with dry toilet paper only after each bowel movement as this will quickly make the delicate skin sore and unnecessarily uncomfortable.

After each bowel movement, drink a half to full cup of freshly boiled hot water. Record your observations of each bowel movement as soon as possible afterwards while it is fresh in your memory.

Write it in your journal or type it directly into your online tracker. Make it a point to record each bowel movement right away so that you have an accurate record.

Usually, urges for bowel movements will appear every 20 to 60 minutes. On average, expect to have one to two movements per hour. There may also be a peak period where you experience four to five for an hour and then it slows down. This is normal and you'll need to pay attention to fluid consumption so that you continue to drink at least one half cup of hot water after each bowel movement.

The biggest risk during this stage is dehydration. Careful monitoring of fluid intake will largely prevent this. A total of two to four liters of freshly boiled hot water should be consumed over the course of the entire day. Remember to record fluid intake as well so you have an accurate total at the end of the day.

It is normal to feel more tired and exhausted as the day progresses. However, you cannot fall asleep at any point during the day. If it helps, get up and walk around every 15 to 30 minutes, play enjoyable music, or put something on the TV to create background noise and activity. You can sit comfortably with legs extended on the couch, sofa or bed for as long as it does not cause you to feel sleepy.

End of purgation

At some point between 3 pm and 6 pm, you will likely start to notice bowel movements slowing down to once per hour or less. Additionally, you'll probably notice a feeling of hunger starting to gently increase. When you believe bowel movements have likely stopped, take a warm shower. Do not apply any oil before or after.

After showering, dry off and get dressed in warm clothes. Drink more hot water, and observe your feelings of hunger. If bowel movements have almost certainly stopped and you are definitely hungry, go ahead and have your first recovery meal (Recovery meal #1, congee water) with the flavoring specified in the recipe. Note that these flavors should be subtle yet enjoyable and satisfying.

It is best to eat this between 5 pm and 8 pm , and then rest. You can go to bed as early as 7 pm and lie down, relax and fall asleep.

Stage 5, Recovery

Recovery stage to restore healthy *doṣhas* (*paśhchat karma*), with therapeutic meals (*samsarjana krama*)

Purpose and duration

Immediately following purgation day, the body is typically exhausted and weak from the reduction en masse via waste materials and fluids. The core digestion and metabolism (*agni*) is also weakened due to the stress of the entire procedure.

Stage 5: Recovery, is designed to reestablish core digestion and metabolism (*agni*) by gradually building and strengthening it using a very specific, structured sequence of meals. This phase of rehabilitation meals is called *samsarjana krama*. Additionally, Stage 5 allows for the integration of all aspects and outcomes of Complete Virechana so that you can move into your ideal, healthy diet and lifestyle.

The density and flavoring progressively increases to spark digestion and metabolism over a set number of meal times. This is determined based on the outcome of the previous stage.

Your Āyurveda Āchārya will provide a clear meal plan and instructions on how to prepare the density and flavoring for each meal throughout Stage 5. Depending on how many bouts of bowel movements you had during Stage 4, your rehabilitation diet may require 3 to 7 days.

Beyond this very specific diet, expect to reintroduce foods slowly and scientifically. Introduce no more than three foods or ingredients each day for two to four weeks following Stage 5.

Routine and activities

Throughout Stage 5, expect to continue to rest and recuperate. Do not plan any activities that require physical or mental energy. Do not engage with friends or family except for short periods with calm, easy conversations.

Your daily routine will look very similar to the previous stages. Continue to wake up naturally at or before sunrise and go to bed when you feel tired around 7 pm or later. You must be asleep by 9:30 pm or 10 pm at the absolute latest.

If you wake up very early and cannot go back to sleep, do not force yourself to sleep again, otherwise it risks damaging the hormonal system (specifically healthy cortisol function). Instead, get up when you feel sufficiently rested or that you cannot go back to sleep again. Do your morning hygiene routine and drink 1 to 2 cups of freshly boiled hot water.

If you are awake during the hours of 2 am to 6 am and you fell asleep around 8 pm the night before, know that this is a very good sign that the internal functioning of the body is resetting and strengthening. During these very early hours of the morning, engage yourself in any mental activities that will help you achieve your life goals. This can include reading, writing, journaling, meditation, memorizing, chanting, affirmations, visualizations, gratitude or other types of practices. The goal is to bolster your sense of individuality and strengthen it by building knowledge, skills and emotional stability that will help you achieve your goals.

Around sunrise, put all of these activities away, and transition into activities that bring awareness into the physical body. Practice gentle Yoga Āsana, stretching or other movement activities that are comfortable within your current limits. It is imperative that you do not overextend yourself physically during Stage 5, and if you notice that happening, immediately slow down and regulate your breathing or rest. Avoid any activities that raise your heart rate or require you to breathe heavily. Do not do any *prāṇāyāma* exercises that raise the heart or breathing rate.

After gentle activity, you should take a warm to hot shower. Do not perform *abhyaṅga* or use any oil until your Āyurveda Āchārya informs you that you can start. For the first few days of Stage 5, you can also skip a morning shower if you feel too exhausted or weak.

After showering, dress warmly and have your first meal of the day when you feel hungry. Continue to sip on freshly boiled hot water around meal times and throughout the day. If instructed by your Āyurveda Āchārya, you may also include an herbal tea.

During the day, activities will continue to be limited to easy, stress-free things like watching tv, listening to audio books or videos, painting, coloring, arts and crafts, music and stretching. Walk around more each day as your energy increases. Towards the end of Stage 5 you should expect to start doing gentle body-weight exercises to begin reengaging muscles to start rebuilding strength.

Meals

During Stage 5, meals are specifically designed to reinstate digestion and metabolism (*agni*) to a healthy, normal baseline state. It is absolutely imperative that these be followed exactly as your Āyurveda Āchārya instructs. Any deviation from meals during Stage 5 can lead to difficult, painful consequences that can produce physical and mental symptoms or complications.

At the end of the day of Stage 4: Elimination, your Āyurveda Āchārya will calculate your results of bowel movements and assess your outcomes to determine your meal plan for Stage 5. Be sure to write down exactly what you should have for each meal using the planning tools in the Appendix or your online tracker.

For most, a three-meal per day schedule will be recommended. Typically this means that breakfast is around 7am to 8 am, lunch is around 11am to 12 pm and dinner is around 5 pm. In some exceptional cases, four meals per day may be required, however it is not ideal. No snacking at all is allowed during this stage.

Make sure that you eat enough at each meal to last you about 4 hours until the next meal. If you are not able to eat a sufficient quantity, let your Āyurveda Āchārya know. There may be adjustments to the recipe that will help make it easier for you to eat a little more.

During Stage 5, meals will start off as the water of cooked congee initially and gradually increase in density over a few days. The base of the congee is usually rice but may be a different grain as needed. Flavors will also be introduced gradually in a specific order.

Standard recipes for Stage 5 are included in the Appendix of this book. Be sure to read through all of these well before your actual procedure. You should even practice cooking congee at least once before starting Virechana so that you understand the recipes and requirements. When in doubt about any meals, take pictures and show your Āyurveda Āchārya for confirmation.

At the beginning of Stage 5, check your stock of fresh vegetables and ingredients on hand. If needed, get fresh items delivered so that you have good quality ingredients to use as the meals and flavors build up each day.

Throughout Stage 5, you will continue to meet with your Āyurveda Āchārya daily for assessments and a review of your progress. In many cases, signs and symptoms will continue to appear throughout this stage. These are mostly related to being exhausted, weak and still recovering from Stage 4, and this is completely normal. In some cases, signs or symptoms of underlying pathology may appear as the body is now able to address it in a cleaner state.

Be sure to discuss any signs or symptoms that you notice with your Āyurveda Āchārya. It is always your responsibility to clearly state what you're experiencing so that you can discuss it and make any adjustments if needed.

Post-virechana

Regeneration period to arrest ageing (*rasāyana* or *śhamana*), with formulations (*auṣhadha*)

Purpose and duration

The post-virechana regeneration period can last anywhere from 40 to 180 days, depending on the individual's choices and diligence in following healthy routines, diets and habits. Immediately after Complete Virechana, the physical body is exceptionally clean. Much of the physical and metabolic waste that has been interfering with optimal physiological function has been eliminated.

The body has literally and figuratively undergone an oil change which has profound, systematic benefits like clearing major and minor channels, and flushing the liver and other digestive organs. The weeks to months that follow this deep cleanse and reset are a prime opportunity for promoting the regenerative capacity of the body, stabilizing the mind and strengthening one's complete being. When done well, this supports longevity with a high quality of life and minimal disease.

Your Āyurveda Āchārya can prepare a plan for you to use Āyurvedic formulations (*auṣhadha*) that promote ongoing doṣha stabilization and normalization (*śhamana*) through pacification, reduction or promotion of strength of one or more *doṣhas*. It is important to note that regular follow-ups are required during this period to maximize benefits and avoid relapse or complications.

Additionally, you will continue to work with your Āyurveda Āchārya to understand all of the ongoing changes and improvements that occur well after Complete Virechana. If any signs or symptoms indicate deeper layers of pathology, you may consider additional rounds of Medical Pañcha Karma as appropriate. These are generally recommended each year during middle age (30 to 70 years) to prevent disease and promote a strong foundation of health, immunity and overall satisfaction and capability throughout life.

Appendix 1: Glossary

Āyurvedic Sanskrit Term	Short Definition
abhyaṅga	A full-body oil massage that may be performed on one's own or by trained, same-sex therapists in a Pañcha Karma facility
abhyantara sneha (or snehana)	Internal lubrication produced by oral consumption of fatty media such as ghee or oil
āma	Internally-generated waste products that form due to incomplete or incorrect digestion
auṣhadha	Āyurvedic formulations that are capable of producing a specific outcome based on a targeted line of action; always referred to as Āyurvedic medicines in India
Āyurveda Āchārya	An Āyurvedic Medical Doctor who has completed a minimum of 5.5 years of training from an accredited institution and is licensed to practice Āyurvedic medicine
Āyurvedic medicine	The complete healthcare system of health maintenance and disease management which originated in and around India
bahir parimarjana	The classification of external therapies which includes full body oil massage, steam heat, poultice, pouring treatments and various massages
bāhya sneha (or snehana)	External lubrication produced by application of oil to the entire body and scalp, followed by steam heat and shower
basti	Therapeutic enema; the third (and fourth, according to one classification) of the five Medical Pañcha Karma procedures; the two types of basti include nirūha (emulsion enema) and anuvāsana (oil enema)
congee, or kañji	Rice gruel or soup made from a single type of rice cooked in a large quantity of water until the rice grains break down and soup becomes slightly thick

Complete Pañcha Karma	Five therapeutic procedures used in Āyurvedic medicine to eliminate accumulated waste products (as *doṣhas*) from the physical body
dīpana	Stimulation of the appetite to increase intake capacity
doṣha	Physiological regulator that produces health or wastes leading to disease; operates based on inputs of diet, lifestyle, activities, genetics, environment, etc; includes three *doṣhas* of the physical body, *vāta*, *pitta* and *kapha*
koṣhṭha	The gastrointestinal tract (GIT) from mouth to anus; classified into three types based on functional state
Medical Pañcha Karma	See Complete Pañcha Karma
Mini Pañcha Karma	Adaptations of Complete Pañcha Karma that allow certain procedures to be performed immediately, without the preparatory stages of lubrication and mobilization
nasya	Therapeutic nasal instillation; the fourth (or fifth, according to one classification) of the five Medical Pañcha Karma procedures
pāchana	Digestive stimulation to improve processing, metabolism and conversion of consumed food and drink
Pañcha Karma	The group of five procedures in Āyurvedic medicine that are designed to target and eliminate accumulated, latent *doṣhas* from the physical body
Pañcha Karma Lite	Application of select manual therapies for spa, beauty and relaxation purpose; not related to the therapeutic effects of Complete or Medical Pañcha Karma; generally, a misnomer where treatments would be better grouped under the *bahir parimarjana* classification
paśhchat karma	The third stage of recovery in Medical Pañcha Karma which restores *doṣhas* to their healthy, normal functioning levels
pradhāna karma	The second stage of operation in Medical Pañcha Karma which eliminates the *doṣhas* from their nearest route of exit

pūrva karma	The first stage of preparation in Medical Pañcha Karma which prepares the *doṣhas* for elimination
rakta mokṣhaṇa	Therapeutic blood-letting; the fifth of the five Medical Pañcha Karma procedures
rasāyana	Regeneration or regenerative therapeutics; a specialty branch of Āyurvedic medicine that restores and regenerates the body to its optimal state; ideally performed after correct elimination therapy using Medical Pañcha Karma
rūkṣhaṇa	Producing a drying effect in the body
sadyo virechana	Literally, "sudden elimination"; therapeutic purgation without preparatory lubrication and mobilization
samsarjana krama	Rehabilitation diet after elimination in Medical Pañcha Karma
śhamana	Stabilization or normalization of one or more of the *doṣhas* in the physical body or mind; practically achieved via pacification, reduction or promotion of the *doṣhas*
śhiro abhyaṅga	Application of oil to the scalp followed by head massage
śhodhana	Elimination of one or more of the *doṣhas* from the physical body
sneha pāna	Oral intake of fats, usually ghee or oil
Svastha Āchārya	An Āyurvedic Health Coach
svedana	Heat treatment that induces sweating; may be performed using various types of equipment or methods
vamana	Therapeutic emesis; the first of the five Medical Pañcha Karma procedures
virechana	Therapeutic purgation; the second of the five Medical Pañcha Karma procedures

Appendix 2: Recipes

Preparation meal #1

Use the following recipes, according to your instructions, for preparation meals.

1. Recovery meal #4, Thick Congee
2. Recovery meal #5, Rice and Lentil Soup (no oil)
3. Recovery meal #6, Rice and Lentil Soup (with oil)
4. Recovery meal #7, Meat Soup

Or, follow your specific instructions.

Recovery meal #1, Congee Water (*Maṇḍa*)

This is the first meal allowed after the elimination stage of Virechana because it is the lightest and easiest to digest. Depending on the strength of the digestive power, it may digest in 2 - 4 hours.

1. Use ½ cup of aged basmati rice, or another low-glycemic index rice. Most of the rice will not be eaten, but is required to thicken the congee water. This entire portion can be enough for 2 servings.
2. Prepare the rice by washing it thoroughly. Rub and squeeze the grains through the hand. Empty the water, and repeat 2-3 times until the water runs clear and any sediment has washed away.
3. Add 8-10 times of clean, cool water to the washed rice.
4. Do not add any spices or anything else.
5. Put the pot on the stove on medium to high heat.
6. Bring to a full boil, then reduce the heat to allow it to gently boil.
7. The pot can be half covered to allow it to cook more easily. Watch for bubbling and boiling over, and adjust or remove the cover if necessary.
8. Adjust the heat as needed through the cooking process.
9. Stir occasionally to make sure grains are moving easily and not stuck together.
10. Continue to add boiled water to the pot to keep the overall water level high. Do not allow the congee to become thick at any point.
11. When most of the grains have broken down and the consistency of the water is thicker, the congee should be ready. The final pot should have at least 3 cups of congee water (liquid) remaining. If it is lower than 3 cups, add more water and simmer for a few minutes.
12. Remove from heat, and stir well.
13. Serve in a glass measuring cup so you can measure how much you are consuming. Start with a 1-cup portion, and see how filling it is before eating any more. The final amount and proportions of rice grains and congee water in the measuring cup should be as follows:
    a. rice grains - no more than 25% or ¼ cup mark

b. congee water - 75% proportion, water should reach the 1 cup mark

14. Add the following garnish
    a. 1 pinch of pink, Himalayan crystal salt
    b. Stir well and dissolve the salt completely. The final serving should not taste salty or leave any coating on the teeth or in the mouth.
15. If instructed, add these additional items for garnish
    a. about 10 drops of fresh lime
    b. about 5 drops of ghee
    c. ¼ teaspoon or less of raw cane sugar
    d. Stir well and dissolve the salt and sugar completely. The final serving should not taste salty, sour or sweet. Instead, the flavors should blend together and taste almost milky or like freshly baked bread.
16. Do not add any other ingredients to the final serving.

Recovery meal #2, Thin Congee (*Peya*)

This is the second meal allowed after the elimination stage of Virechana. It is slightly heavier and more nourishing than the first recovery meal of congee water. Depending on the strength of the digestive power, it may digest in 3 - 4 hours. Wait at least 4 hours before eating after this meal.

1. Use ½ cup of aged basmati rice, or another low-glycemic index rice. Some of the rice will not be eaten, but is required to thicken the congee water. This entire portion can be enough for 2 servings.
2. Prepare the rice by washing it thoroughly. Rub and squeeze the grains through the hand. Empty the water, and repeat 2-3 times until the water runs clear and any sediment has washed away.
3. Add 8-10 times of clean, cool water to the washed rice.
4. Do not add any spices or anything else.
5. Put the pot on the stove on medium to high heat.
6. Bring to a full boil, then reduce the heat to allow it to gently boil.
7. The pot can be half covered to allow it to cook more easily. Watch for bubbling and boiling over, and adjust or remove the cover if necessary.
8. Adjust the heat as needed through the cooking process.
9. Stir occasionally to make sure grains are moving easily and not stuck together.
10. Continue to add boiled water to the pot to keep the overall water level high. Do not allow the congee to become thick at any point.
11. When most of the grains have broken down and the consistency of the water is thicker, the congee should be ready. The final pot should have at least 3 cups of congee water (liquid) remaining. If it is lower than 3 cups, add more water and simmer for a few minutes.
12. Remove from heat, and stir well.
13. Serve in a glass measuring cup so you can measure how much you are consuming. Start with a 1-cup portion, and see how filling it is before eating any more. The final amount and proportions of rice grains and congee water in the measuring cup should be as follows:

a. rice grains - no more than 50% or ½ cup mark
b. congee water - 50% proportion, water should reach the 1 cup mark

14. Add the following garnish
    a. 1 pinch of pink, Himalayan crystal salt
    b. Stir well and dissolve the salt completely. The final serving should not taste salty or leave any coating on the teeth or in the mouth.
15. If instructed, add the following garnish
    a. Additional ¼ teaspoon pink, Himalayan crystal salt
    b. freshly squeezed juice of ¼ slice of lemon
    c. Stir the lemon juice in well and dissolve the salt completely. The final serving should taste pleasantly sour and salty. The flavors should blend together well and neither should overpower the other.
    d. If needed, adjust the flavors by adding small amounts of one or the other until is reaches a pleasant, well-combined final taste.
16. Do not add any other ingredients to the final serving.

Recovery meal #3, Medium Congee (*Vilepī*)

This is the third meal allowed after the elimination stage of Virechana. It is slightly heavier and more nourishing than the second meal of thin congee. Depending on the strength of the digestive power, it may digest in 4 - 5 hours. Wait at least 4 hours before eating after this meal.

1. Use ½ cup of aged basmati rice, or another low-glycemic index rice. Some of the rice will not be eaten, but is required to thicken the congee water. This entire portion might be enough for 2 servings.
2. Prepare the rice by washing it thoroughly. Rub and squeeze the grains through the hand. Empty the water, and repeat 2-3 times until the water runs clear and any sediment has washed away.
3. Add 8-10 times of clean, cool water to the washed rice.
4. Do not add any spices or anything else.
5. Put the pot on the stove on medium to high heat.
6. Bring to a full boil, then reduce the heat to allow it to gently boil.
7. The pot can be half covered to allow it to cook more easily. Watch for bubbling and boiling over, and adjust or remove the cover if necessary.
8. Adjust the heat as needed through the cooking process.
9. Stir occasionally to make sure grains are moving easily and not stuck together.
10. Continue to add boiled water to the pot to keep the congee soupy. It should not become very thick.
11. When most of the grains have broken down and the consistency of the water is thicker, the congee should be ready. The final pot should have at least 2 cups of congee water (liquid) remaining. If it is lower than 2 cups, add more water and simmer for a few minutes.
12. If instructed, add 2 handfuls of freshly washed arugula (rocket) leaves, stir, and simmer for 1 - 2 minutes, or until the leaves are fully cooked. Do not overcook.
13. Remove from heat, and stir well.

14. Serve in a glass measuring cup so you can measure how much you are consuming. Start with a 1-cup portion, and see how filling it is before eating any more. The final amount and proportions of rice grains and congee water in the measuring cup should be as follows:
    a. rice grains - no more than 75% or ¾ cup mark
    b. congee water - 25% proportion, water should reach the 1 cup mark
15. If instructed, add the following garnish
    a. ½ teaspoon raw cane sugar
    b. Or 1 pinch of pink, Himalayan crystal salt
    c. Stir well and dissolve the sugar or salt completely.
16. If using arugula leaves and sugar, the final serving should taste bitter and slightly sweet.
17. If using salt only, the final serving should not taste salty or leave any coating on the teeth or in the mouth.
18. Do not add any other ingredients to the final serving.

Recovery meal #4, Thick Congee

This is the fourth meal allowed after the elimination stage of Virechana. It is slightly heavier and more nourishing than the third meal of medium congee. Depending on the strength of the digestive power, it may digest in 4 - 5 hours. Wait at least 4 hours before eating after this meal.

1. Use ½ cup of aged basmati rice, or another low-glycemic index rice. Some of the rice will not be eaten, but is required to thicken the congee water. This entire portion will be enough for 1 - 2 servings.
2. Prepare the rice by washing it thoroughly. Rub and squeeze the grains through the hand. Empty the water, and repeat 2-3 times until the water runs clear and any sediment has washed away.
3. Add 8-10 times of clean, cool water to the washed rice.
4. Add the following spices
    a. ½ teaspoon dry ginger powder or freshly ground ginger root
    b. ½ teaspoon coriander powder
    c. ¼ teaspoon black pepper powder
    d. any other recommended spices
5. Put the pot on the stove on medium to high heat.
6. Bring to a full boil, then reduce the heat to allow it to gently boil.
7. The pot can be half covered to allow it to cook more easily. Watch for bubbling and boiling over, and adjust or remove the cover if necessary.
8. Adjust the heat as needed through the cooking process.
9. Stir occasionally to make sure grains are moving easily and not stuck together.
10. Continue to add boiled water to the pot to keep the congee soupy. It should not become very thick.
11. When most of the grains have broken down and the consistency of the water is thicker, the congee should be ready. The final pot should look like normal congee in thickness.
12. Remove from heat, and stir well.

13. Serve in a glass measuring cup so you can measure how much you are consuming. Start with a 1-cup portion, and see how filling it is before eating any more. The final amount and proportions of rice grains and congee water in the measuring cup should be as follows:
    a. rice grains - around 90% or almost at the 1 cup mark
    b. congee water - water should reach the 1 cup mark, or go just over
14. Add the following garnish
    a. ¼ teaspoon pink Himalayan crystal salt
    b. If instructed, 1 - 2 teaspoons of freshly washed, chopped cilantro leaf
15. Stir well and dissolve the salt completely.
16. The final serving should taste slightly hot and spicy. If it is not spicy at all, add small amounts of black pepper powder or red chili powder to taste.
17. Do not add any other ingredients to the final serving.

Recovery meal #5, Rice and Lentil Soup, no oil (*Akṛta yūṣha* + protein)

This is the fifth meal allowed after the elimination stage of Virechana. It is the first meal after congee and introduces regular, cooked rice with lentil or dal soup. Depending on the strength of the digestive power, it may digest in 4 - 6 hours. Wait at least 4 hours before eating after this meal.

Soup preparation

1. Use ½ cup yellow lentils or split yellow moong beans (with or without the green shell).
2. Prepare by washing thoroughly and rinsing several times, or until the water runs clear.
3. Add 5 - 6 times more water for cooking.
4. Add the following spices, or follow your specific instructions.
    a. ½ teaspoon dry ginger powder or freshly ground ginger root
    b. ½ teaspoon coriander powder
    c. ¼ teaspoon black pepper powder
    d. any other recommended spices
5. Put the pot on the stove on medium to high heat.
6. Bring to a full boil, then reduce the heat to allow it to gently boil.
7. The pot can be half covered to allow it to cook more easily. Watch for bubbling and boiling over, and adjust or remove the cover if necessary.
8. Adjust the heat as needed through the cooking process. If foam appears on the surface while cooking, it can be removed and discarded.
9. Stir occasionally to make sure everything is moving easily and not stuck together.
10. If the soup becomes too thick, add more freshly boiled hot water and stir well.
11. The soup is ready when the lentils or beans have completely broken down and the consistency is medium thick. If the soup is too thick, add more freshly boiled hot water, stir and cook gently for a few more minutes.

12. Remove from heat, and stir well.
13. Serve the amount for the meal in a separate bowl, then add the following garnish
    a. ¼ teaspoon pink Himalayan crystal salt
    b. about 10 drops of freshly squeezed lime
    c. Optionally, 1 - 2 teaspoons of freshly washed, chopped cilantro leaf
14. Stir well and dissolve the salt completely.
15. The final serving should taste flavorful, without a single, pronounced flavor.
16. Do not add any other ingredients to the final serving.
17. If having the soup with rice, mix the soup with the rice and eat both together.

Rice preparation

1. Use ¼ to ½ cup of aged basmati rice, or another low-glycemic index rice, depending on your desired portion size.
2. Prepare the rice by washing it thoroughly. Rub and squeeze the grains through the hand. Empty the water, and repeat 2-3 times until the water runs clear and any sediment has washed away.
3. Add enough water to cover the rice by about ⅛ to ¼ inch, or 1 - 2 cm. To further reduce the glycemic effects of the cooked rice, use more water and drain it after the rice is cooked.
4. Allow the rice to soak for 10 minutes before cooking.
5. If using a rice cooker, press the button and wait for the rice to finish cooking.
6. If cooking on the stove, bring to a full boil, then reduce the heat to allow it to gently boil.
7. Cook gently with the cover on or slightly open to prevent bubbling.
8. Adjust the heat as needed through the cooking process.
9. When the rice grains are fully open and soft, the rice is ready.
10. If required, drain the excess cooking water immediately.
11. Keep the rice in the pot, covered and hot until ready to serve.

Recovery meal #6, Rice and Lentil Soup, with oil (*Kṛta yūṣha* + fat)

This is the sixth meal allowed after the elimination stage of Virechana. It is the first meal that introduces oil or fat. For vegetarians, this is the final meal in the recovery diet. It may be eaten for several meals in a row at the end of the process.

Depending on the strength of the digestive power, it may digest in 4 - 6 hours. Wait at least 4 hours before eating after this meal.

Soup preparation, part 1

1. Use ½ cup yellow lentils or split yellow moong beans (with or without the green shell).
2. Prepare by washing thoroughly and rinsing several times, or until the water runs clear.
3. Add 5 - 6 times more water for cooking.
4. Add the following spices, or follow your specific instructions.
    a. ½ teaspoon turmeric powder
    b. any other recommended spices
5. Put the pot on the stove on medium to high heat.
6. Bring to a full boil, then reduce the heat to allow it to gently boil.
7. The pot can be half covered to allow it to cook more easily. Watch for bubbling and boiling over, and adjust or remove the cover if necessary.
8. Adjust the heat as needed through the cooking process. If foam appears on the surface while cooking, it can be removed and discarded.
9. Stir occasionally to make sure everything is moving easily and not stuck together.
10. If the soup becomes too thick, add more freshly boiled hot water and stir well.
11. The soup is ready when the lentils or beans have completely broken down and the consistency is medium thick.

12. Remove from heat, stir well, and keep covered until ready to use in part 2.

Soup preparation, part 2

1. In a separate fry pan, skillet or wok with a well-fitting cover, add about 2 tablespoons of fat (olive oil, coconut oil or ghee, according to your instructions).
2. Optional: If using mustard seeds, heat the pan, spread the fat evenly and heat the fat to smoke point. Quickly add ½ teaspoon mustard seeds into the hot oil or ghee, and cover immediately. Shake the pan gently and allow the seeds to pop, then immediately reduce the heat or remove from heat (if using a cast iron pan). Add any remaining spices in order, being careful to avoid burning them.
3. In the heated pan, add the following spices to the oil or ghee
    a. ½ teaspoon freshly ground ginger root
    b. ½ teaspoon coriander seed powder
    c. ¼ teaspoon black cumin seed or regular cumin seed
    d. optional, 1 - 2 pinches of red chili flakes or powder
    e. optional, 4 - 6 fresh curry leaves
4. Adjust the heat so that the spices do not burn. Stir and cook the spices evenly. They can cook and burn quickly and suddenly. Watch for any sudden popping of water droplets that can splash hot ingredients.
5. As soon as the spices smell properly cooked
    a. Optional - add ½ sliced sweet, yellow onion and cook until translucent
    b. Optional - add a single vegetable and cook until soft, like celery, broccoli, peas, kale, chopped green beans, or any Indian gourd.
    c. Then add the boiled lentil or moong bean soup. If at the correct temperature, this will bubble and splatter as it hits the pot.
6. Stir well and bring to a simmer.

7. Cook the entire pot together for 3 - 5 minutes, or until mixed to the proper consistency. If too thick, add small amounts of freshly boiled hot water and mix well.
8. While simmering, add salt, taste as needed, and adjust.
9. When it tastes complete, remove from heat.
10. Serve in a separate bowl, and garnish.
    a. about 10 drops of freshly squeezed lime
    b. Optionally, 1 - 2 teaspoons of freshly washed, chopped cilantro leaf
11. Stir well and dissolve the salt completely.
12. The final serving should taste flavorful, without a single, pronounced flavor.
13. Do not add any other ingredients to the final serving.
14. If having the soup with rice, mix the soup with the rice and eat both together.

Rice preparation

1. Use ¼ to ½ cup of aged basmati rice, or another low-glycemic index rice, depending on your desired portion size.
2. Prepare the rice by washing it thoroughly. Rub and squeeze the grains through the hand. Empty the water, and repeat 2-3 times until the water runs clear and any sediment has washed away.
3. Add enough water to cover the rice by about ⅛ to ¼ inch, or 1 - 2 cm. To further reduce the glycemic effects of the cooked rice, use more water and drain it after the rice is cooked.
4. Allow the rice to soak for 10 minutes before cooking.
5. If using a rice cooker, press the button and wait for the rice to finish cooking.
6. If cooking on the stove, bring to a full boil, then reduce the heat to allow it to gently boil.
7. Cook gently with the cover on or slightly open to prevent bubbling.
8. Adjust the heat as needed through the cooking process.
9. When the rice grains are fully open and soft, the rice is ready.
10. If required, drain the excess cooking water immediately.
11. Keep the rice in the pot, covered and hot until ready to serve.

Recovery meal #7, Meat Soup (*Māṁsa rasa*, fat + protein)

This is the seventh and final meal in the recovery process after cleansing the body for non-vegetarians. It should be cooked in the morning on the day of use and be eaten for several meals with plain rice, couscous or a small amount of freshly toasted bread.

Depending on the portion size, it will digest in 4 - 6 hours. Wait at least 4 hours after this meal before eating your next meal.

Any single type of meat can be used with this recipe. Do not use fish or seafood.

- Whole chicken
- Lamb cut, with bone
- Beef cut, with bone
- Pork cut, with bone
- Venison cut, with bone

Preparation instructions

1. Prepare the cut of meat. Wash, and if needed cut into small or medium sized pieces, and remove all excess fat and slime.
2. In a large stock pot, heat 3 - 4 tablespoons of olive oil. Coat the bottom of the pot evenly.
3. When the oil is hot and almost at smoke point, add the following, one at a time, stirring until each is cooked. Or, follow your specific flavoring instructions.
4. 1 - 3 teaspoons freshly ground ginger root
5. 1 - 3 cloves of garlic (optional)
6. 1 - 3 bay leaves
7. ½ to 1 flat teaspoon turmeric powder
8. When all spices are moderately cooked, add 1 large, diced, sweet yellow onion.

9. Optionally, add chopped celery and diced celery root. Stir and coat in oil, and cook until all ingredients are lightly browned.
10. Add the meat. Keep the temperature on low so that it does not cook too quickly so that it becomes tough.
11. Stir well, coat in the oil and spices, and continue to stir and cook until lightly browned.
12. While the meat is cooking, sprinkle salt and black pepper on it and continue to stir and cook.
13. Add boiling hot water to cover all ingredients well. Mix thoroughly and allow to simmer.
14. Cook covered or partially covered on low until the meat is cooked all the way through and the vegetables are soft and broken down.
15. Add salt, black pepper to taste.
16. Serve and optionally garnish with any one of cilantro leaf, parsley leaf, basil leaf, etc.
17. Allow the remaining portion to cool and immediately store it in the refrigerator.
18. When reheating, take only the portion to be consumed and reheat it. Do not save reheated portions for later use.
19. Eat with freshly cooked rice, couscous or a small amount of bread, whole wheat pita, or other simple grain.

Appendix 3: Supplies

Time Pass

What's time pass? It's a fun phrase used in India for anything that passes the time.

	Must have	Nice to have
Time pass	Easy reading materials, books	Legos
	Self-development books, materials, practices	Board games
	Electronic devices (laptop, iPad, phone)	Cards
	Journaling materials	Dice
	Meditation or Yoga practices	Sewing, crocheting, knitting
	Any spiritual practices, reading material	Drawing, coloring or painting
	Pleasant movies	
	Music	
	Pictures	
	Easy instruments to play	

Personal supplies

Be sure to have enough on hand for the entire procedure, or plan to do laundry midway.

	Must have	Nice to have
Personal supplies	Comfortable clothing made from all-natural fabric that is breathable and warm	Hair dryer, especially for longer hair
	Socks and warm footwear	Additional warm slippers
	Bath towels, face cloths	Favorite pillow(s)
	Wide-toothed comb, hair clips or hair ties	
	Gentle soap, preferably fragrance-free	
	Gentle shampoo, preferably fragrance-free (no conditioner needed)	
	Comfortable sheets made from all-natural, breathable fabric	
	Nail clipper	
	Trimmer, razor	
	Toothbrush, toothpaste, floss	
	Feminine hygiene products (pads, tampons, menstrual cup, period underwear)	

General supplies

It is recommended to have all items on hand to make the process more safe comfortable.

	Must have	Nice to have
General supplies	Water filter	Stainless steel flask to keep hot water
	Electric kettle, drinking cups	Cheesecloth or plain, clean cloth for straining
	Glass measuring cups (Pyrex, heat proof) with metric measurements in 10 milliliter increments from 50ml to 200ml	Bidet for toilet (installed or portable)
	Small to medium sized pots for cooking individual servings	Portable steam tent where the head remains outside of the heat
	Oven mitts, kitchen towels, cooking utensils, tableware and utensils	Finger Pulse Oximeter, (SpO2) Blood Oxygen Saturation Monitor
	A blender, juicer or mortar and pestle	Thermometer
	Digital scale for kitchen with metric measurements in 1 gram increments	Body weight scale
	Measuring spoons	
	Blood pressure apparatus	

Pantry items and ingredients

All pantry items must be on hand before starting.

Required materials and ingredients	Approximate quantity	
Aged basmati rice, or other low-glycemic rice	½ to 1lb (½ kg)	☐
Couscous	1 small box	☐
Quinoa	2 cups (250 gm)	☐
Pinto beans, red or yellow lentils, or whole chicken	Few servings	☐
Cracked wheat or bulgur	Few servings	☐
Whole wheat flour or atta flour	Few servings	☐
Moong dal (split or whole)	Few servings	☐
Oil (olive, coconut or sesame)	4 cups (1 liter)	☐
Pink, Himalayan crystal salt	4 tsp (20 gm)	☐
Raw cane sugar	2 tsp (10 gm)	☐
Ginger powder	8 Tbs (100 gm)	☐
Coriander seed or powder	8 Tbs (100 gm)	☐
Black pepper powder	2 tsp (10 gm)	☐
Fenugreek seed or powder	2 tsp (10 gm)	☐
Turmeric powder	2 tsp (10 gm)	☐

Hing powder	1 tsp (5 gm)
Bay leaves	About 10
Cumin seed, and/or black cumin seed	2 tsp (10 gm)
Red chili flakes or powder	2 tsp (10 gm)
Black mustard seeds	2 tsp (10 gm)

Fresh foods

Plan to have these on hand at the start and re-stocked in Stage 3 or 4 if needed.

Required fresh foods	**Approximate quantity**
Fresh ginger root	2 – 3 inch piece
Lime	1 – 2
Meyer's lemon (if available)	1 – 2
Garlic	1 bulb
Fresh cilantro leaves (coriander)	1 bunch
Fresh parsley leaves (any kind)	1 bunch
Fresh basil leaves	1 bunch
Fresh curry leaves (if available)	1 bunch
Celery stalks	1 bunch

Celery root (celeriac)	1 bulb	☐
Arugula (rocket)	1 – 2 bunches	☐
Kale (any kind)	1 – 2 bunches	☐
Yellow or sweet onions (small)	2 – 3	☐
Broccoli, asparagus, green beans	1 – 2 servings, of choice	☐
Apples (sweet, not sour, medium size)	5 – 6	☐
Ghee	2 – 3 tablespoons	☐

Āyurvedic formulations

Confirm with your Āyurveda Āchārya before purchasing any formulations.

Formulations required	**Quantity**	
Avipatti churna (powder)	10 packets	☐
Trivrilleham (paste)	1 bottle	☐
Gandharvahasthadi kashayam (liquid)	1 bottle	☐
Gandharvahasthadi tailam (oil)	1 bottle	☐
Triphala powder	100 gm	☐
Haritaki powder	10 gm	☐
Ashta churna (powder)	1 bottle	☐
Kshirabala taila (oil for abhyaṅga)	2 bottles	☐

Additional formulations required

Appendix 4: Mini Virechana Records

Planning

Mini Virechana	Number of days	Start date	End date
Stage 1 Preparation	1 to 5 days, or more		
Stage 2 Elimination	1 day (rarely 2 days)		
Stage 3 Recovery	3 to 5 days		
Post-Mini Virechana Regeneration	2 to 4 weeks		

Stage 1: Mini Virechana Preparation

Date: ________________________		**Mini Virechana Preparation** **DAY 01**
Activity or event	Time	Details and observations
Local sunrise time		
Wake up, clean up, bowel movement		
Oil massage, steam bath, shower, rest		
Morning formulation		
Digestion assessment		
First meal		

Treatment(s)		
Second meal		
Evening formulation		
Third meal		
Activities and significant events		
Bedtime		

Date: ______________________________		**Mini Virechana Preparation** **DAY 02**
Activity or event	Time	Details and observations
Local sunrise time		
Wake up, clean up, bowel movement		
Oil massage, steam bath, shower, rest		
Morning formulation		
Digestion assessment		
First meal		

Treatment(s)		
Second meal		
Evening formulation		
Third meal		
Activities and significant events		
Bedtime		

Date: ______________________		Mini Virechana Preparation DAY 03
Activity or event	Time	Details and observations
Local sunrise time		
Wake up, clean up, bowel movement		
Oil massage, steam bath, shower, rest		
Morning formulation		
Digestion assessment		
First meal		

Treatment(s)		
Second meal		
Evening formulation		
Third meal		
Activities and significant events		
Bedtime		

Date: ______________________________		Mini Virechana Preparation DAY 04
Activity or event	Time	Details and observations
Local sunrise time		
Wake up, clean up, bowel movement		
Oil massage, steam bath, shower, rest		
Morning formulation		
Digestion assessment		
First meal		

Treatment(s)		
Second meal		
Evening formulation		
Third meal		
Activities and significant events		
Bedtime		

Date: ______________________________		Mini Virechana Preparation DAY 05
Activity or event	Time	Details and observations
Local sunrise time		
Wake up, clean up, bowel movement		
Oil massage, steam bath, shower, rest		
Morning formulation		
Digestion assessment		
First meal		

Treatment(s)		
Second meal		
Evening formulation		
Third meal		
Activities and significant events		
Bedtime		

Stage 2: Mini Virechana Elimination

Date: ______________________		**Mini Virechana POOP DAY**
Activity or event	Time	Details and observations
Local sunrise time		
Wake up, clean up, bowel movement		
Oil massage, steam bath, shower, rest		
Poop medicine		
Shower, Recovery meal, bedtime		

Poop num	Time	Mini Virechana Details
1		
2		
3		
4		
5		
6		
7		
8		
9		
10		
11		
12		
13		
14		
15		
16		

Stage 3: Mini Virechana Recovery

Date: ______________________		**Meal Planner**	**Mini Virechana Recovery Day 01**
Meal	Density	Flavors	
1			
2			
3			

Date: ______________________	**Mini Virechana Recovery**	**Day 01**
Activity or event	Time	Details and observations
Local sunrise time		
Wake up, clean up		
First meal		
Second meal		
Third meal		
Bedtime		

Date: ______________________		Meal Planner	Mini Virechana Recovery Day 02
Meal	Density	Flavors	
1			
2			
3			

Date: ______________________	Mini Virechana Recovery	Day 02
Activity or event	Time	Details and observations
Local sunrise time		
Wake up, clean up		
First meal		
Second meal		
Third meal		
Bedtime		

Date: ______________		Meal Planner	Mini Virechana Recovery Day 03
Meal	Density	Flavors	
1			
2			
3			

Date: ______________________	Mini Virechana Recovery	Day 03
Activity or event	Time	Details and observations
Local sunrise time		
Wake up, clean up		
First meal		
Second meal		
Third meal		
Bedtime		

Date: ______________________		Meal Planner Mini Virechana Recovery Day 04
Meal	Density	Flavors
1		
2		
3		

Date: ______________________	Mini Virechana Recovery	Day 04
Activity or event	Time	Details and observations
Local sunrise time		
Wake up, clean up		
First meal		
Second meal		
Third meal		
Bedtime		

Date: ______________		Meal Planner	Mini Virechana Recovery Day 05
Meal	Density	Flavors	
1			
2			
3			

Date: ______________________		Mini Virechana Recovery **Day 05**
Activity or event	Time	Details and observations
Local sunrise time		
Wake up, clean up		
First meal		
Second meal		
Third meal		
Bedtime		

Appendix 5: Complete Virechana Records

Planning

Complete Virechana	Number of days	Start date	End date
Stage 1 Preparation			
Stage 2 Lubrication	3 to 7 days		
Stage 3 Mobilization	3 days		
Stage 4 Elimination	1 day (rarely 2 days)		
Stage 5 Recovery	3 to 7 days		
Post-virechana Regeneration	2 to 6 months		

Optional travel plan	Number of days	Start date	End date
Travel to facility			
Rest period to adjust circadian clock			
Total time for Virechana	10 to 20 days		
Rest period to prepare for travel			
Travel to return home			
Post-virechana Regeneration	2 to 6 months		

Stage 1: Complete Virechana Preparation

Meals	Recommendations	Explanation

Activities	Recommendations	Explanation

Self-care treatments	Materials needed	Method

Other instructions	Materials needed	Method

Date: ______________________________	Complete Virechana Preparation	DAY 01
Activity or event	Time	Details and observations
Local sunrise time		
Wake up, clean up, bowel movement		
Oil massage, steam bath, shower, rest		
Morning formulation		
Digestion assessment		
First meal		

Treatment(s)		
Second meal		
Evening formulation		
Third meal		
Activities and significant events		
Bedtime		

Date: ______________________		Complete Virechana Preparation DAY 02
Activity or event	Time	Details and observations
Local sunrise time		
Wake up, clean up, bowel movement		
Oil massage, steam bath, shower, rest		
Morning formulation		
Digestion assessment		
First meal		

Treatment(s)		
Second meal		
Evening formulation		
Third meal		
Activities and significant events		
Bedtime		

Date: ______________________________________	Complete Virechana Preparation	DAY 03
Activity or event	Time	Details and observations
Local sunrise time		
Wake up, clean up, bowel movement		
Oil massage, steam bath, shower, rest		
Morning formulation		
Digestion assessment		
First meal		

Treatment(s)		
Second meal		
Evening formulation		
Third meal		
Activities and significant events		
Bedtime		

Stage 2: Complete Virechana Lubrication

Date: ______________________	**Complete Virechana Lubrication DAY 01**
Consumed: ______________________	Quantity: ________________

Activity or event	Time	Details and observations
Local sunrise time		
Wake up, clean up, bowel movement		
Drink fat		
During fat digestion		
Shower		

After shower digestion assessment		
First congee		
Activities and significant events		
Additional congee(s)		
Total fluid intake		
Bedtime		

Date: ______________________ Consumed: ______________________		**Complete Virechana Lubrication** **DAY 02** Quantity: ________________
Activity or event	Time	Details and observations
Local sunrise time		
Wake up, clean up, bowel movement		
Drink fat		
During fat digestion		
Shower		

After shower digestion assessment		
First congee		
Activities and significant events		
Additional congee(s)		
Total fluid intake		
Bedtime		

Date: ______________________________ Consumed: ______________________________		Complete Virechana Lubrication **DAY 03** Quantity: ______________________
Activity or event	Time	Details and observations
Local sunrise time		
Wake up, clean up, bowel movement		
Drink fat		
During fat digestion		
Shower		

After shower digestion assessment		
First congee		
Activities and significant events		
Additional congee(s)		
Total fluid intake		
Bedtime		

Date: ______________________ Consumed: ______________________		**Complete Virechana Lubrication DAY 04** Quantity: ________________
Activity or event	Time	Details and observations
Local sunrise time		
Wake up, clean up, bowel movement		
Drink fat		
During fat digestion		
Shower		

After shower digestion assessment		
First congee		
Activities and significant events		
Additional congee(s)		
Total fluid intake		
Bedtime		

Date: ______________________________ Consumed: ______________________________		**Complete Virechana Lubrication DAY 05** Quantity: ______________________
Activity or event	Time	Details and observations
Local sunrise time		
Wake up, clean up, bowel movement		
Drink fat		
During fat digestion		
Shower		

After shower digestion assessment		
First congee		
Activities and significant events		
Additional congee(s)		
Total fluid intake		
Bedtime		

Date: ____________________ Consumed: ____________________		**Complete Virechana Lubrication** **DAY 06** Quantity: ________________
Activity or event	Time	Details and observations
Local sunrise time		
Wake up, clean up, bowel movement		
Drink fat		
During fat digestion		
Shower		

After shower digestion assessment		
First congee		
Activities and significant events		
Additional congee(s)		
Total fluid intake		
Bedtime		

Date: ______________________	Complete Virechana Lubrication **DAY 07**
Consumed: ______________________	Quantity: ________________

Activity or event	Time	Details and observations
Local sunrise time		
Wake up, clean up, bowel movement		
Drink fat		
During fat digestion		
Shower		

After shower digestion assessment		
First congee		
Activities and significant events		
Additional congee(s)		
Total fluid intake		
Bedtime		

Stage 3: Complete Virechana Mobilization

Date: ______________________	**Complete Virechana Mobilization**	**DAY 01**
Activity or event	Time	Details and observations
Local sunrise time		
Wake up, clean up, bowel movement		
Breakfast (only if instructed)		
Oil massage and steam bath		
Shower and rest		

First meal		
Activities and significant events		
Second meal		
Bedtime		

Date: ________________________	**Complete Virechana Mobilization**	**DAY 02**
Activity or event	Time	Details and observations
Local sunrise time		
Wake up, clean up, bowel movement		
Breakfast (only if instructed)		
Oil massage and steam bath		
Shower and rest		

First meal		
Activities and significant events		
Second meal		
Bedtime		

Date: ______________________	Complete Virechana Mobilization	DAY 03
Activity or event	Time	Details and observations
Local sunrise time		
Wake up, clean up, bowel movement		
Breakfast (only if instructed)		
Oil massage and steam bath		
Shower and rest		

First meal		
Activities and significant events		
Second meal		
Bedtime		

Stage 4: Complete Virechana Elimination

Date: ______________________________	**Complete Virechana POOP DAY**	
Activity or event	Time	Details and observations
Local sunrise time		
Wake up, clean up, bowel movement		
Oil massage and steam bath		
Shower and rest		
After shower digestion assessment		

Virechana formulations		
After formulations symptoms and assessment		
Shower		
After shower digestion assessment		
Recovery meal 01		
Total fluid intake		
Rest and bedtime		

Poop num	Time	Details
1		
2		
3		
4		
5		
6		
7		
8		
9		
10		
11		
12		
13		
14		
15		

Poop num	Time	Details
16		
17		
18		
19		
20		
21		
22		
23		
24		
25		
26		
27		
28		
29		
30		

Stage 5: Complete Virechana Recovery

Date: ____________________		**Meal Planner**	**Complete Virechana Recovery Day 01**
Meal	Density	Flavors	
1			
2			
3			

Date: ______________________________		Complete Virechana Recovery Day 01
Activity or event	Time	Details and observations
Local sunrise time		
Wake up, clean up		
First meal		
Second meal		
Third meal		
Bedtime		

Date: ____________________		Meal Planner Complete Virechana Recovery Day 02
Meal	Density	Flavors
1		
2		
3		

Date: ______________________		Complete Virechana Recovery Day 02
Activity or event	Time	Details and observations
Local sunrise time		
Wake up, clean up		
First meal		
Second meal		
Third meal		
Bedtime		

Date: ____________________		**Meal Planner** **Complete Virechana Recovery Day 03**
Meal	Density	Flavors
1		
2		
3		

Date: ______________________________		Complete Virechana Recovery Day 03
Activity or event	Time	Details and observations
Local sunrise time		
Wake up, clean up		
First meal		
Second meal		
Third meal		
Bedtime		

Date: ____________________		Meal Planner	Complete Virechana Recovery Day 04
Meal	Density	Flavors	
1			
2			
3			

Date: ______________________________		Complete Virechana Recovery Day 04
Activity or event	Time	Details and observations
Local sunrise time		
Wake up, clean up		
First meal		
Second meal		
Third meal		
Bedtime		

Date: ______________		Meal Planner Complete Virechana Recovery Day 05
Meal	Density	Flavors
1		
2		
3		

Date: ______________________ **Complete Virechana Recovery Day 05**

Activity or event	Time	Details and observations
Local sunrise time		
Wake up, clean up		
First meal		
Second meal		
Third meal		
Bedtime		

Date: ____________________		Meal Planner — Complete Virechana Recovery Day 06
Meal	Density	Flavors
1		
2		
3		

Date: ______________________________		Complete Virechana Recovery Day 06
Activity or event	Time	Details and observations
Local sunrise time		
Wake up, clean up		
First meal		
Second meal		
Third meal		
Bedtime		

Date: ____________________		Meal Planner	Complete Virechana Recovery Day 07
Meal	Density	Flavors	
1			
2			
3			

Date: ______________________________		Complete Virechana Recovery Day 07
Activity or event	Time	Details and observations
Local sunrise time		
Wake up, clean up		
First meal		
Second meal		
Third meal		
Bedtime		

References

Literature on Āyurvedic medicine and Āyurvedic Medical Pañcha Karma is extensive. Key references are included here for further research. However, this is not an exhaustive reference list of subject material.

Classical literature

Śharmā, R. K., & Dāsha, B. Agniveśha's Charaka Saṁhitā. Varanasi: Chowkhamba Sanskrit Series Office; Reprint Edition. 2016. Cha. Sū. 13/ - 16/, Cha. Si. 1/ - 12/.

Murthy, K. R. Srikantha. Vāgbhaṭa's Aṣhṭāṅga Hṛdayam. Chowkhamba Kṛṣhṇadas Academy, Varanasi. Reprint Edition. 2016. AH. Sū. 16/ - 18/.

Singhal, G.D., et al. Suśhruta Saṁhitā of Suśhruta. Chaukhamba Sanskrit Pratiśhthan, Reprint Edition. 2015. Sū. Chi. 31/ - 34/.

Contemporary literature

Mulay MS. Short term escalating administration of large amount of sneha does not increase blood lipids. J Ayurveda Integr Med. 2021 Jul-Sep;12(3):535-539. doi: 10.1016/j.jaim.2020.05.004. Epub 2020 Jul 28. PMID: 32732172; PMCID: PMC8377170.

Chaturvedi A, Rao PN, Kumar MA, Ravishankar B, Rao N, Ravi M. Effect and Mechanism of Virechana Karma (Therapeutic Purgation) Over Fructose-Induced Metabolic Syndrome: An Experimental Study. J Evid Based Complementary Altern Med. 2016 Jul;21(3):194-201. doi: 10.1177/2156587215596283. Epub 2015 Jul 22. PMID: 26207023.

Chaturvedi A, Nath G, Yadav VB, Antiwal M, Shakya N, Swathi C, Singh JP. A clinical study on Virechana Karma (therapeutic purgation) over the gut flora with special reference to obesity. Ayu. 2019 Jul-Sep;40(3):179-184. doi: 10.4103/ayu.AYU_302_19. Epub 2020 Aug 8. PMID: 33281395; PMCID: PMC7685265.

Pandya M, Donga SB, Dei LP, Thakar AB. Efficacy of Virechana, Triphaladi decoction with processed Guggulu in the management of ovarian cyst - A pilot study. Ayu. 2020 Jul-Sep;41(3):166-172. doi: 10.4103/ayu.AYU_254_19. Epub 2022 Feb 24. PMID: 35370374; PMCID: PMC8966757.

Talekar MT, Mandal SK, Sharma RR. Clinical evaluation of Trivṛta powder (Operculina turpethum Linn.) and Aragvadha Patra Lepa (paste of leaves of Cassia fistula Linn.) in the management of Vicharchika (eczema). Ayu. 2018 Jan-Mar;39(1):9-15. doi: 10.4103/ayu.AYU_45_15. PMID: 30595628; PMCID: PMC6287402.

Rais A, Bhatted S. Clinical study to evaluate the effect of Virechanakarma on serum electrolytes. Ayu. 2013 Oct;34(4):379-82. doi: 10.4103/0974-8520.127719. PMID: 24696575; PMCID: PMC3968700.

Ghosh KA, Tripathi PC. Clinical effect of Virechana and Shamana Chikitsa in Tamaka Shwasa (Bronchial Asthma). Ayu. 2012 Apr;33(2):238-42. doi: 10.4103/0974-8520.105244. PMID: 23559796; PMCID: PMC3611644.

Patil, Vaidya Vasant & Baghel, Madhaw & Thakar, A.B.. (2009). Effect of Snehapana (Internal Oleation) On Lipids: A Critical Review. Ancient science of life. 29. 32-9.

Dissanayake, K.G.C. & SK, Tiwari. (2007). Effect of Snehapana with Virechana Therapy on the Lipid Profile of Patients with Over Weight.

Made in the USA
Monee, IL
08 November 2026

67816241R00129